A BODY WISDOM BOOK

125
128
129

• LIGHT TOUCH FOR OPTIMAL HEALTH •

BODY
WISDOM

Sharon Giammatteo, Ph.D.
Edited by Thomas Giammatteo, D.C.

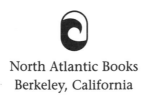

North Atlantic Books
Berkeley, California

Published by
North Atlantic Books
P.O. Box 12327
Berkeley, California 94712

Cover and book design © Ayelet Maida, A/M Studios
Cover art © Inge Eibl
Illustrations in Parts I and II © Inge Eibl; in Part III © Alanna Rosano
Photographs © John Giammatteo
Printed in the United States of America

Body Wisdom is sponsored by the Society for the Study of Native Arts and Sciences, a nonprofit educational corporation whose goals are to develop an educational and crosscultural perspective linking various scientific, social, and artistic fields; to nurture a holistic view of arts, sciences, humanities, and healing; and to publish and distribute literature on the relationship of mind, body, and nature.

North Atlantic Books' publications are available through most bookstores. For further information, call 800-337-2665 or visit our website at www.northatlanticbooks.com.

Substantial discounts on bulk quantities are available to corporations, professional associations, and other organizations. For details and discount information, contact our special sales department.

Library of Congress Cataloging-in-Publication Data

Giammatteo, Sharon
   Body wisdom : light touch for optimal health / Sharon Giammatteo.
   p. cm.
   Includes index.
   ISBN 1-55643-356-5 (alk. paper)
   1. Touch—Therapeutic use. 2. Post-traumatic stress disorder—Alternative treatment. 3. Self-care, Health. I. Title.

RZ999.W45 2001
615.8'22 21; aa05 01-22—dc01
                                                      2001016263

2 3 4 5 6 7 8 9 MALLOY 07 06 05 04 03

Contents

For my sister, Tammy

Foreword

Trauma is not a rare event. It affects millions of individuals, causing tremendous amounts of (unnecessary) suffering. Unfortunately, treatment is often based on victimhood rather than open empowerment and true healing.

Body Wisdom helps to empower individuals in reclaiming the healing resources that are everyone's birthright. It is a deeply moving and personal account of self-awakening and an inspirational tale of Sharon Giammetteo's journey of transforming the traumatic "hand of cards" she was dealt as a child. Beyond this, Sharon presents a series of body-based "energy" exercises to help readers restore their vitality and balance in the aftermath of overwhelming and shaming experiences. These "process exercises" can assist readers in recovering the sense of self and wholeness lost in the wake of trauma.

Sharon Giammatteo is a leading innovator in the field of Physical Therapy. She has pioneered many advanced techniques in rehabilitation medicine. Dr. Giammatteo is widely recognized for these contributions.

In this book, Sharon brings together in simple language her theoretical knowledge of the nervous and other bodily systems with an understanding of the emotional, energetic, and spiritual bodies.

With compassion and clarity, Sharon honors our innate capacity for self-regulation and healing. She gently guides the reader on the pathway to awakening. Read, learn, experience, and heal.

Peter Levine, Ph.D.
Author of *Waking the Tiger: Healing Trauma*
North Atlantic Books, 1997

Acknowledgements

I wish to acknowledge Dr. Inge Eibl, for her illustrations which have provided enormous impact.

My respect and appreciation to John Giammatteo, whose photography is such a gift.

My gratitude and appreciation to my daughter, Ayelet, for her diligence and love, for her support and encouragement. Without her, this book would not have happened.

My appreciation to Matt Walstatter, for his exceptional editing of the book.

My appreciation to my colleague Heather Mulcahey, who contributed her time and effort for the photographs.

Many thanks to my colleagues who have used this work, Neurofascial Process, for their own healing, to benefit family, friends, and clients.

Many, many thanks to my clients whose healing was my stimulus to write *Body Wisdom*.

My love and smiles to Nim, Ayelet, and Amir, my children whose blessings continue to be such a gift. They have supported me and the development of this work for so many years.

To my husband, Tom, I give credit for the birth of this book. His love, attention to detail, encouragement, and integrity brought this book to fruition.

Thank you all and so many others,

Sharon

Introduction

Over many years of professional study and practice I developed Integrative Manual Therapy^{SM}, a comprehensive system of healing for body, soul, and spirit. It is based on principles of "manual medicine" and was developed over three decades of work in a wide range of bodywork and psychotherapeutic methods. I truly believe that Integrative Manual Therapy is the most thorough system of healing of this kind in practice today, for it has grown from the study of the emotional and spiritual meaning of virtually every detail of human anatomy and functioning.

Neurofascial Process^{SM}, which this book is about, is a subdivision of Integrative Manual Therapy that you can perform on yourself without the aid of trained practitioners, physicians, or therapists of any kind. It is an extremely simple method for healing every kind of physical and emotional problem. It does not require special skills—only patience, hope, and persistence, and a minimal amount of understanding in order to orient the work and give it direction. Everything you need to know to use Neurofascial Process is contained in this book.

Since the early '80s I have taught Integrative Manual Therapy and Neurofascial Process with my husband, Thomas Giammatteo, in seminars and workshops across the United States.

In this book I tell my personal story—how I came to the knowledge that allowed me to develop these methods, and how, through their practice, I have come to experience a measure of fulfillment and continuing inner growth that, judging from my early life, should have been almost impossible. I am telling my story in order to use my own experience as an object lesson in how we all can achieve self-fulfillment through the release of repressed memories and emotions and by learning to live fully in the present. The exercises explained in this book have been my own basic healing practice for over thirty years. I have spent literally thousands of hours working with them, and I can honestly say that I owe my own healing to what I learned through them. They have been the means for integrating everything else I have come to understand.

The exercises involve placing one's hands over specific parts of one's body for extended periods of time, and simply "being-with" what comes to consciousness while doing so. Anyone can begin to apply them immediately. There are no contraindications. My own professional work has involved correlating an enormous amount of neuroanatomical information with the intimate insights I have gained through performing these processes, but it is in no way necessary to have any of this knowledge in order to use them for self-discovery and self-healing.

Though I claim to be the originator of Integrative Manual Therapy and Neurofascial Process—and it certainly is the case that I myself fleshed-out the methods it employs through my own study, practical investigations, and intellectual efforts—the truth is that its guiding insights came to me through a series of extraordinary experiences: the recurring presence of an inner guiding "voice" that has been with me since I was a little child. The voice came to me unexpectedly and unsought when I was suffering terribly at the hands of members of a violent and malevolent household. Its counsel made it possible for me to survive intolerable conditions of childhood sexual abuse, and, as I grew older, taught me how to heal myself through performing the very processes that I share in this book. It has guided my study and practice as a healer to the present day, and I am offering its wisdom to the readers in the hope that they will be able to find in it a source of spiritual nourishment and personal growth.

This book has three parts. In Part I, I introduce Neurofascial Process by telling the story of how it was developed. It is my own story, and in many ways it is quite shocking. I tell my story in detail so that it might have the greatest impact, but some readers may feel uncomfortable hearing about these unpleasant things. If you do, you may choose to skim over the earlier chapters.

Part II is presented most of all for those who wish to recover from severe psychoemotional trauma. But the beauty of this part of the book is that even if you do not have any history of profound emotional problems, you will find opportunities for growth and development. I present there the basic ideas necessary to understand how to work with

Neurofascial Process, namely, the *Six Bodies* that everyone has and that make up the deep structure of the Self. Healing work involves becoming aware of our personal issues in relation to these bodies. I also present in Part II the Process Centers that are used in healing work and to which the specific healing methods that will be presented in Part III refer. You should familiarize yourself with these ideas and reread these sections when you need to refresh your memory.

Part III presents an entire system for self-healing, including easy-to-perform exercises useful in healing whatever problem you are suffering from, whether it is a sprained ankle, mild or severe low back pain, abdominal cramps, headaches, or problems with major organs such as the heart, liver, kidney, and so forth. It also presents exercises for emotional and stress-related problems.

It is possible to use these methods in conjunction with whatever other healing practices or medical treatments you are employing. If you are using aspirin or other pain relievers to deal with chronic or acute pain, you don't have to stop doing so. But you may find that after applying these methods you will no longer need them. If you have been suffering from chronic pain that your doctor said you simply would have to live with—don't despair! Don't give up. Try the exercises recommended here and keep working with them. They are very easy to perform, but they may take a lot of time before they begin to be profoundly effective. At the same time keep exploring your options—even beyond the exercises in this book and the kinds of treatments you have been receiving. There is never any need for hopelessness and despair. Today there are so many noninvasive and nonaggressive healing methods appearing all the time.

There are no limitations on the use of Neurofascial Process exercises. If you are bedridden, you can apply them while in bed. If you are not a very disciplined person and watching television is your main form of relaxation—you can work with them while watching television! This work can be performed at home, in the office, at school, in hospitals, in emergency rooms, in cars, airplanes, trains, and buses. I can't think of a setting where it would be wrong to use them.

Though the instructions in this book are for self-healing, the same methods can be applied to you by others, or by others to you. You will see that some of the instructions suggest that you welcome the assistance of friends and loved ones in placing their hands over Process

Centers. This way many centers can be treated together and in relation to one another. The hands that heal you do not necessarily have
to be your own. Conversely, you can use your hands to apply Neurofascial Process to others. If your son or daughter or spouse or parent is
ailing, you can treat them. You don't have to be a self-designated
"healer" with a special calling or special gifts in order to help others
to heal themselves. The methods are available to all.

A few final remarks about how to apply the methods. Though I call
these recommendations "exercises," "methods," and "treatments" inter-
changeably, they are really possibilities for self-exploration. For instance,
I recommend various lengths of time for placing the hands in various
positions. These should be taken as suggestions, not scientific recipes.
The idea is that when something feels to you as though it is working,
keep going! And if it doesn't feel like it is working, be sure you have
given it enough time so that it can have a chance to start to work. It
takes a long time for a person to get sick. It takes lot of work with self-
healing to recover. You could continue for months, treating yourself
for an hour or so a day. You cannot over treat yourself, and in any case,
you will heal in your own time.

The Journey of Transformation to Recall, Recovery, and Neurofascial Process

Within Part I is an historical perspective explaining how this book came about. Many parts of the story are not pleasant; I tell it because perhaps others have similar stories. Whether you, the reader, wish to consider this portion of the book fact or fiction is your choice.

The purpose of this book is *not* to tell my own story. Part I is simply meant to give perspective to the techniques presented in Parts II and III. Please don't put this book down because the first part makes you sad. Go to the techniques. Learn the work. Use this approach to start healing your own mind and body. Skip ahead to the low back pain protocol, or to the stomachache protocol, or to the headache protocol. Above all, this book is meant for your healing.

CHAPTER 1

Early Childhood

The recliner was old and ragged, with ripped seams and stuffing sticking out of the cushions. It sat in one corner of our living room, which was really too small to hold both the chair and our couch comfortably. The combination of the clutter, the size of the house, and the way my family behaved made it feel more like a cage than a house. Sometimes, when I was growing up, I feared that the walls of that living room were closing in on me, suffocating me. Other times, I wished that they would get it over with.

As the old man stood up, the chair let out a groan, as if it was glad to be free, at least temporarily, from the burden of his overweight frame. I listened as he walked into the kitchen and opened the refrigerator. He pulled another red and white can from the top shelf, and I winced involuntarily when I heard him crack it open. I knew that I was in trouble. At the age of four, I didn't know what was in the cans. I didn't even know what beer was. Words like rape, sodomy, and torture meant nothing to me. But I knew the sound of a can of Budweiser opening. And I knew that if I heard it enough times in a row, I was in for a very long night.

My step-grandfather, we called him Zadie, walked from the small kitchen area back into the living room. Even though I was in one of the three upstairs bedrooms, I could hear every noise he made. The sound carried through our house, a small split-level made smaller by the number of people packed into it and the horrible things that they did to each other. I shared this house with my sisters, my brother, my father, my mother, her mother (who had married Zadie after divorcing her first husband), and my mother's two half-sisters, both of whom were mentally retarded.

"Karen, get over here!" Zadie slurred at me. His voice carried throughout the entire house, and I could hear him clearly from my bed. I didn't move though, except to pull the blanket tighter over my head. He would come find me soon enough. I had counted at least eight cans opened so far. Perhaps he would drink one or two more before I heard the awful thud of his feet as he trudged up the stairs, perhaps not.

"I said get over here!" he repeated, sounding meaner than usual.

I pulled the covers tighter, praying in a soft whisper for something, anything, to keep him from coming into the room I shared with my sisters. "Please God, don't let him come up here. Make him fall down. Make him get sick. Make him die. Just don't let him come into this room. Please." I hardly noticed the tears streaming down my face.

Zadie stood up and returned to the kitchen yet again. He opened another can of beer, and I heard him walk past his smelly old chair without sitting down. He continued up the stairs, through the hallway and into my room, where he stopped in the doorway.

I didn't take my head out from under the covers. I didn't have to. I knew exactly what he looked like standing there above me. I knew the red hue of his face and his misshapen nose, the result of a life where his only true companions were beer and whiskey. I knew the exact size of the bald spot that he used to try to hide by combing the rest of his white hair across it, a feat now impossible because he had so little hair left. I knew that his navel was visible because his filthy white undershirt never covered all of his fat stomach. I knew he was wearing greasy pants that he would soon be unbuttoning. But not yet.

"You come when I call you!" he snarled, ripping the blanket off of me. I looked up just in time to see the back of his gnarled, arthritic hand as it landed full force across my face. "Do you understand?... Answer me!"

I understood all too well, but the only response I could muster was a sob, and this wasn't good enough for Zadie, who wound up and let loose with another backhand. "Get up," he shouted, "I'll teach you to listen." He jerked me out of bed, ripped off my pajamas, and threw me on the floor. Then he unbuckled his leather belt and pulled it out from around his waist. He wrapped the side with the buckle around his fist and began whipping me. Blows landed all over my small body. My screaming and crying succeeded only in arousing him further, and he switched ends of the belt, hitting me with the large metal buckle instead.

After what seemed like an eternity, the beating stopped. Through my sobs, the only sound I could hear was his loud, rheumatic breath. All I could do was lie there with my face buried in the carpet. Please let this be all. Please let it be over, I thought. But when I finally summoned the courage to open my eyes and look up through the tears, I saw that it was not over, not even close. Zadie was standing over me with his pants around his ankles and his erect penis in his hand. He grabbed me by the throat and threw me onto the bed. "All right you little bitch," he said, spreading my tiny, frail legs with those dirty, disgusting hands. "This is what happens to bad girls." He shoved a finger inside me, and when I screamed, he slapped me again. "Shut up, you little cunt!"

He sat on my chest and I closed my eyes as he started hitting me in the face, alternating blows between the back of his hand and his penis. I tried to shut off my mind, or go to a different place. I tried to think of something else. Anything else. Then, as he slid down off of my chest and penetrated me, I heard laughter. Not the innocent giggles of schoolgirls, but perverse, demented, evil laughter. I looked up and saw my two half-aunts standing in the doorway, cackling like witches as their father brutally beat and raped me. And then everything went black.

• • •

I grew up in a cold, dark house. We used a coal burner all year round, but it couldn't cut through the frigid atmosphere. There was little access to daylight, but nobody in the household could tell. We were a family without sunshine. In its place was intense fear.

As we grew, most of the time we were oblivious to the physical, emotional, and sexual abuse that occurred daily. The memories were tucked away into the nooks and crannies of our house and our minds, for what we hoped would be forever. But we paid a high price to repress those horrors. Burying my past made me feel as though a large part of me was missing, and this had a profound impact on the rest of my life. Nobody in my family had any idea that we might eventually reach a point of recall, where all of the memories, all of the pain, would resurface. None of us realized that at some point we might remember, and that this would be the key to our recovery.

When I began to recall, I remembered the pain, the abuse, and the terror. And because I remembered, I was able to heal. But I had to go through a great deal, inside and outside of that house, before I was able to recover. I went through a long period of silence, cut off from other people, from any concept of God, from myself.

I repressed my memories during the days, and they found expression only in my nightmares. They were stored away until I reached the age of recall, as if some part of me decided to keep them away from me until I was ready to handle them. So it was not until much later in my life that I began to remember the tragedies of my childhood. One of the great discoveries of my life is that lessons learned are often nothing more than past memories recalled. And that is why we must recall—in order to learn life's lessons.

No life is entirely miserable, and I can smile as I remember happy times: singing with my sister, birthdays and anniversaries, the deep connections that we made with one another. Like other young girls, I played with dolls. When the time came, I went to school and did my homework. And I played piano and other musical instruments.

I don't know exactly when Zadie began beating and raping my sisters and me, but I know that by the time I was three he had begun to molest me, and he may have started when I was even younger than that. And once he started, he didn't let up. We were attacked constantly, and not just by Zadie. My father was physically abusive, and my aunts and their boyfriends abused me both physically and sexually. There were incidents of torture, involving not only sexual and physical assaults, but weapons as well. These were interspersed with daily incidents of rage, terror, and fear, many of which I remembered. The most tragic incidents I forgot. Until I was able to recall.

When I was four years old, I walked in on Zadie molesting my older sister. He was on top of her, cursing at her, and she was crying and screaming for him to stop. I ran at Zadie, hitting him with as much force as my four-year-old muscles could muster. I must have seemed like a gnat buzzing around his ear. But a gnat can be awfully annoying, and he turned his attention from my sister to me. As he got up off of my sister, I turned and ran for the stairs. With Zadie close at my heels, I jumped over the second-floor railing, landing flat on my back on the wood floor below.

At that point I had the first of three near-death experiences that I have faced, each similar to those described by countless others. I saw a tunnel engulfed in rays of white light, and somehow I knew that if

I walked down that tunnel I would be free of all of the misery of my life. I wanted desperately to walk down that tunnel, to leave Zadie and my aunts and the rest of my family behind forever.

As I started down the tunnel, I heard a voice. I can't pinpoint any specific characteristics of the voice—whether it was male or female, loud or soft, even what language it was speaking. In fact, I can't really be sure that it was a voice at all. But it was so authoritative, so wise and all-knowing, that it is tempting to believe that it was the voice of God. And I believe that it was. In retrospect, I am also certain that the voice came from inside me, that it was as much a part of me as my fingers are. More so, in fact. This has led me to the belief that every individual soul is an expression of God, a manifestation of a higher power that binds the universe, that is the universe.

"Turn back," said the voice. "You still have work to do." I was stunned. I wanted more than anything to walk down that tunnel. But somehow I knew that the voice was right. Sensing my conflict, knowing how torn I was, the voice told me to leave my house when I awoke. "Go as far as necessary," it said, "in order to forego your present and fulfill your mission. You will return when the time is right."

All of this sounded like a pretty tall order for a four-year-old of limited means, but the voice continued. "You do not necessarily have to escape physically. Not yet. You can escape into the future. You can plant seeds now that will bloom later. In the mean time, you must tend the garden. If the present is painful, then live in the future. Focus on the excitement and anticipation of the future, and you will never know the pain of the present. Later, when you are strong enough, independent enough, you will recall the suppressed thoughts and emotions. You will be aware of the pain and the trauma, but with a new appreciation for the lessons learned. You will use these memories to heal yourself, and you will become a conscious, enlightened individual, a force to be reckoned with. And I will always be there to guide you, because I am you."

I woke up with a broken back and damage to my aorta, the body's most important artery. More importantly, I awoke with new insight and a greater sense of my own well-being. How can a four-year-old comprehend the complicated existential messages that I heard from God, my soul? I can only assume that I processed them at some unconscious, intuitive level. But somehow I understood that I could overcome the pain. I was too young to physically run away, but I could escape for the time being by focusing on the future, by making my present moment tomorrow rather than today. I awoke to find my life, the life I had left just moments before, a little less painful. My eyes were opened to a joyful future.

CHAPTER 2

Later Childhood and Adolescence

During the early years of my life, my cries for help went unanswered. My father, an uneducated man, could best be described as ignorant of the world in general and of the difficulties my siblings and I faced. He was abusive as well, though not to the extent that Zadie was, so I couldn't look to him for help. My mother and grandmother almost certainly suffered the same abuse that my sisters and I did at the hands of Zadie, and whether it was because they feared him, or because they feared their own memories, they didn't pay me any heed. And as for my aunts, they were as much a part of the problem as Zadie was.

One night when I was six years old, around the time that my brother was born, the family was forced to face the issue. Zadie was raping my sister that night, and he was being particularly brutal, even by his standards. I had learned long ago that trying to stop him would only mean that I was next. Besides, what could a six-year-old girl do to a grown man anyway? But on this night something inside me snapped. The pain of years of torture and abuse welled up inside me, and each of my sister's blood-curdling shrieks reached deeper into my soul than the one before it. The screams were not just her pain. They were my own as well. And they were tearing me apart as they got louder and louder.

Finally, no longer able to sit and listen, I got up and went onto the front porch, where I saw a Louisville Slugger baseball bat leaning against the side of the house. Maybe this will stop him, I thought, as I picked up the bat. I went back into the house and, as quietly as I could, I climbed the stairs and padded down the hall. When I reached the door to our bedroom, I saw Zadie's grotesque naked form on top of my sister's tiny frame, beating her and swearing as he raped her. I crept up behind him, being extra careful not to make a sound, although he was so engrossed in what he was doing that I doubt he would have heard me if I had shouted his name.

When I got right behind him, I lifted the bat and swung it as hard as my small arms were capable of. He screamed as the pine came crashing down on the back of his head, opening a bloody gash. I swung the bat again, and he turned around just in time to watch it crash into his nose and forehead. Zadie was shouting a stream of obscenities, my sister was shrieking, and through my tears I could see that blood (from Zadie and my sister) was everywhere, but I kept hitting him. I wanted the abuse to stop, the terror to end. And something inside told me that the more times I swung the bat, the greater my chances of achieving that goal.

I don't remember how many times I hit him, or how or why I stopped swinging the Louisville Slugger. The next thing I do remember is the chaos and commotion of paramedics taking Zadie away and police officers trying to figure out what I had done and why. Although I didn't kill Zadie that night, I came awfully close. And when the paramedics wheeled him out of the house, it was the last time that he ever crossed our threshold. He spent the rest of his life in a veteran's hospital for the mentally ill. I don't know how badly I injured him, how much longer he lived, or how he eventually died. All I know is that when he left the house that night, he left my life for good. And for that I am thankful.

With Zadie gone, the abuse didn't stop. My aunts were two sick, sadistic women. They were mentally retarded, and Zadie abused them as he abused my sisters and me. This proved to be a horrible combination, as evidenced by the way they treated me. They were merciless. On one occasion, my Aunt Sarah stabbed me in the groin area with a butcher's knife.

And then there were their boyfriends. My aunts often served as our babysitters. Both were extremely promiscuous, and they had men over to the house whenever they could, especially when my parents were out. I remember one of my Aunt Sally's boyfriends, a big burly man named Steve with dark hair and a long beard. One night when I was about ten years old, my parents went to dinner and Steve came over. He and my aunt were drinking and he started kissing her on the couch in front of me. Thinking that they wouldn't notice, I got up to go to my room.

"Wait a minute," Steve said to me as I began to climb the stairs. "Just where do you think you're going?"

"Upstairs to my room," I answered.

"No you're not," he said. "You just sit back down on that couch." I stood motionless, unsure of what to do. "I said sit down!" he shouted.

I returned to the couch, at which point he turned his attention back to my aunt. They kissed some more, and he began unbuttoning her dress, touching and fondling her breasts. I got up slowly, hoping that he would be more interested in my aunt than he was in me, but as I started up the stairs a second time I heard Steve's voice again. "I thought I told you to stay on that couch." He got up, grabbed me by the shoulders and dragged me down the stairs and back into the living room. I tried to resist him but he was far too strong. He threw me down on the couch, ripped my dress off of me, and raped me, while my aunt sat on the couch next to me, her dress only half on, squealing with delight.

There were more abuses, more traumas, and more horrible incidents. My aunts' boyfriends continued to rape me until I was about eleven years old. Why did they stop then? Perhaps they saw that I was growing up and feared that people might begin to take me seriously. Or maybe my aunts just stopped dating rapists. I don't know. But even though I grew up in that awful home, it was around that time that I began to have a life outside of it. I was popular and successful in school, a star at both basketball and volleyball. I joined different groups and clubs, and I had friends and boyfriends. But none of them ever visited my house. I did everything I could to move my life away from it.

How was I able to accomplish all of this worldly success? I can honestly say that I do not know. I wasn't there. My present was so horrible that I lived entirely in the future.

At night I alternated between insomnia and nightmares. It was as if when I fell asleep, all of the memories that I had shut out, all of the abuses and traumas, were being churned, processed and stored so that later I could recall them. I spent my days living in the promise of the future, and my nights filling my memory banks with the horrors of the present and wrestling phantoms of the past. But I experienced the wonders of the world as I perceived it: the wonders of the future. As a result, I was all smiles and carefree innocence. And this is the major paradox of my young life. The pain was so deeply repressed that I could feel only joy. People commented on this—an elementary school report card described me as "exuberant, almost to a fault." They could see a happiness in my eyes that sprang from the depths of my soul.

While I was able to lock up the worst of my experiences in a dusty trunk somewhere far in the back of the cobweb-filled attic of my memory, I still had to live in that house. And for as much as I focused on the future, I could not entirely escape the discontent and the rage of the other inhabitants of the house. So more and more I dedicated myself to other pursuits outside the house—sports, music, and friends. Unfortunately, friendships held their own perils for me. One of the cornerstones of friendship is sharing, and what could I share? Not my home, filled with anger and abuse, insomnia and nightmares. Not my family, with the yelling and screaming, the rage and the hatred. And certainly not myself. I was disconnected from my present, living through the promise of a future that I didn't clearly understand. How could I share myself when I didn't know who I was? I listened and I learned and I did my best to be a friend to others around me. But nobody could really be my friend. I wouldn't allow it. As I continued to repress my past and my present, I became less and less grounded, to my friends, to my family, to myself. That was the price that I paid for my joy: the inability to experience my present or to share it with others.

It was only my faith, faith in the voice I had heard as a young child, faith in a destiny as yet unfulfilled, which got me through my childhood and adolescence. I trusted that voice more than I trusted anything else in the universe. I knew somehow that it was the voice of God, the voice of my soul, the voice of eternity. And that voice had told me unequivocally that there was to be great happiness in my future. So I lived increasingly in the future, and I felt only joy, even though it meant losing contact with both my internal and my external worlds.

CHAPTER 3

Israel

In retrospect, it's hard to imagine that I stayed in that house as long as I did. But the kind of abuse that I suffered, whether it is repressed or not, leaves a child scared. Despite my various successes in school, sports, and music, I was not at all confident in my identity or my capabilities. I had spent most of my young life alternating between the roles of sex toy and punching bag, and on some deep level I wondered: if this is how my family treats me, what can I expect from the rest of the world? It was almost as if the more pain that I suffered in that house, the more attached to it I became and the harder it was for me to leave. I was also concerned about my brother and my sisters. I didn't want to abandon them. And I believed in the importance of education. I felt that without it I didn't stand a chance of surviving and succeeding, but it was more than simply a survival expedient. Education was a symbol to me of my desire to transcend the circumstances that I was born into and move beyond the horrors of my past. Running away from home would have meant dropping out of high school, which would have shattered my dreams of going to college.

When I did finally graduate from high school, I was ready to go, and I decided to get as far away from that house and its inhabitants as I possibly could. I went to Israel, ostensibly to attend college, and I began a new life there—a new school, new friends, new love. As my orientation shifted, almost imperceptibly, away from the future, I began, ever so slightly, to regain the present. This, I later learned, is the very first step toward recall. In order to deal with my past I would first have to learn to participate in the present.

My first boyfriend in Israel died in combat during the Six Day War. Nevertheless, I finished college, got married, and had three beautiful children. Through them I learned of the love between a mother and her children. I was finally able to see, firsthand, what a happy childhood looks like. But as I turned toward the present for the first time in many years, my memories began to surface. They were hazy and sporadic at this point, but there was no denying them. This caused me a great deal of stress, something that I had avoided by repressing my memories. As the process of recall proceeded, my past gradually started to intrude upon my present, causing hatred, fear, and anger. I was not yet ready to relive the past. It was not yet time for memory to help heal me. Confused, I decided to change my present, both physically and emotionally. Only later would I learn the significance of the connection between the two. I returned to America, and in the process I returned to the future.

But in order to live in the future, I was forced to forego the present with my children. I did not physically abandon them. I continued to live with them and to take care of them, but because I was living in the future, I wasn't really there. It was as if they became memories to me, and I talked about them often. The short time that I had spent with my children, conscious of the present, became everything to me. I was living in the future and in an isolated segment of my past simultaneously.

Although they were never beaten, molested, or abused, my children began to experience some of my past. I was present in the house, yet they did not have a mother who was conscious of the present, who was truly living, to share their lives with. They searched for me. They knocked at my door. They called out to me, forgiving me for everything without even realizing that it was necessary. Where was I? I was with them in the past, without them in the present or future.

Return to the U.S.

When I returned to America, I began working as a physical therapist. I spent my days helping people to heal injuries and overcome pain. It was ironic, because by then, that is how my memories were manifesting themselves—as physical pain. I had back pain, neck pain, chest pain, leg pain, arm pain, and headaches. I hurt constantly, and I hurt all over. I could no longer escape through sports and music because I no longer had the capacity for those activities. I hurt too much. In the terminology of my field, I was somaticized: all of the memories that I had repressed and all of the emotions that I had not dealt with had hardened into dense energies throughout my body, causing pain, dysfunction, and disability.

I continued the facade of my life, playing the roles of wife, mother, and professional as well as I could manage. But I was reaching a turning point. I remembered the voice that had guided me as a young child, and the promises of a future filled with joy and hope. And I slowly began to realize that the process of discovering that joy would begin within me. The first step was to deal with my own pain. And so I began to face the pain, to seek answers. I did not seek in a conventional manner. In a sense, I already knew where I would find what I was looking for—inside of myself. The voice had promised to show me the way, and that voice was simply a manifestation of something that was at once a part of me and entirely beyond me. It gradually dawned on me that if I simply faced the present and looked my pain dead in the eye, the answers would come to me. The only way to find what I was looking for was to search by not searching, and that is exactly what happened. Instead of asking questions directly, I sought change by simply being, and the answers that I needed were right where I knew that they would be, in the voice of the universe, the voice of my soul.

Once I began to embrace the present, to deal with my pain instead of repressing it, amazing things began to happen. I learned a great deal, both worldly knowledge and the wisdom of the soul. This enabled me to grow and evolve. But most importantly, I was able to heal. My life was transformed from an empty existence based on ignoring the present and avoiding pain, to a fulfilling life grounded in love and joy. I attained this transformation by gaining insight from God, my soul, and the world around me and applying that knowledge in the form of specific techniques which had a profound impact upon my life.

I did not create this knowledge or invent these techniques. I am not the only person who understands them or can teach them. Many people do both. And I am certainly not the only person who can benefit from them. I offer my story because anyone who has suffered can heal themselves the same way that I have. It is a long, slow process, but it is highly rewarding. The many benefits include freedom from emotional and physical pain, the ability to live in the present, and more meaningful connections with friends and family. But the real reward lies in the rediscovery of the Self, its place in the world, its connection with everything in the universe and its relationship to, and identity with, God.

CHAPTER 5

Facing the Past:
The Six Bodies

I had already gone to school to heal others, and I was finally ready to heal myself. As I began to embrace this process I needed knowledge, and that knowledge came to me through the same voice that has guided me throughout my life. It spoke to me on various occasions: in my dreams, when I meditated, and while I was in the hypnogogic state—that no man's land between sleep and wakefulness. Sometimes the voice came randomly, while I was driving my car or treating a patient. I listened and I learned.

Over a period of several years I learned of the six "bodies" that we each have. I learned of them through conversations with the higher power that I will refer here to simply as "the Voice." As I discovered the existence of each body, I was able to come in conscious contact with these bodies, the Voice, and Self. I have encapsulated these conversations in order to explain the bodies more concisely.

"The wonders of the universe," the Voice told me one day, "are the bodies of Self, for the manifestation of the *soul*. Your first body, the one you are most familiar with, is the *physical body*. Ideally, its many parts work together as an integrated whole, providing the power that drives your other bodies for an entire lifetime. All of the energies of God's universe run through your skeleton, providing the power that your tissues and organs need. The physical body can be a vehicle that allows Self to perform its tasks effortlessly. But it requires constant input from the world around it to maintain its energy."

As a physical therapist this was not really news to me. But then I learned of the *Emotional Body,* and its connection with the physical body. "You have an Emotional Body as well," the Voice told me, "which emits and controls the energies of your emotions. It involves the physical body tissues, and requires a specific energy flow through those tissues. This Emotional Body's expression is based on a sort of electrochemistry. When you feel an emotion, a wave of energy travels along the tissues, causing them to release chemicals known as peptides, which further the effects of the emotional process. Perception of emotions depends on the Emotional Body, as well as the structures in the physical body which interface with the Emotional Body and which are used to sense and process emotions. By emotions I mean joy, happiness, sorrow, grief, fear, anger, and others. When you perceive emotions, when you truly feel them throughout your physical body, you are able to learn from them. You gather more information, and produce more emotional energies that enable you to work and play. Personal growth ultimately depends on the proper functioning of the Emotional Body."

Next the Voice taught me about my *Spiritual Body*. "Your Spiritual Body is your direction, your purpose, your drive, your meaning. You have a Spiritual Body for the sake of God. It is the avenue of the universe, representing involvement in *practice*. " Practice, I learned, refers to an individual's daily, soul-directed activities. "Your Spiritual Body is your own part in the meaningful drama which never ends, but continues in the cycle of death and life, death and life. It is your brother, your sister, and your friend; your past, your present, and your future; your connection, your being and your true process. Your Spiritual Body causes your heart to yearn for more, much more, allowing you to reach above and beyond your present existence. This body is inside you, surrounding you, and it pervades every part of all of your other bodies. You *are* because you are the Spiritual Body. Being means being your Spiritual Body. Every day. Every night. The state of being is the state of being the Spiritual Body."

I knew that eventually, when my own process had progressed far enough, my task would be to teach others what I learned, so that they could use this information to heal themselves. But it was also intuitive and difficult to comprehend. I wondered how I could communicate this knowledge to others.

"We all communicate in the same language," answered the Voice one day, before I even realized that I had posed the question. "We speak our thoughts of tomorrow today, of today yesterday. We converse with friends we have yet to meet through the *collective unconscious*. All of this occurs when thought is produced in our minds by the *Mental Body*, an energetic structure that is larger than words, greater than languages, more profound than thoughts. It is the body of life's foreplay, the energy that can guide us to God with the greatest of ease, or send us to hell with delusions and fantasies. The Mental Body may communicate with or without us. It can define and it can diffuse. It can protect and it can attack. It can offer understanding and it can create chaos. The Mental Body has the ability to formulate a plan, and along with the other bodies, it can implement that plan. It interfaces with the Emotional Body, as well as with the Spiritual Body. It can be your friend or your enemy. It is the language of love as well as the conduit of hate. Be *with* the Mental Body. Be *in* the Spiritual Body. *Ask permission* of the physical body. Be *affected* by the Emotional Body."

As the years progressed and my insight increased, I heard about my *Personal Body.* "Your Personal Body is a body like any other, with a beginning and an end. It is the energies within you that fulfill your duty to your Soul. Passions pervade your Personal Body, bringing strength of character and softness in traits. You express your being through your Personal Body by manifesting your personality traits, which are unique to you. They are your energetic structure, with a form and substance of their own. You have the potential to be more or less than any single characteristic. Your mission is to find your own balance. Your purpose coincides with finding a presence for your Personal Body, and *simply being* is a good way to achieve that goal. That is, being in the now allows your Personal Body to express itself, with all of its characteristics and all of its passions."

I learned that we all determine our person at any given point in time, but often we don't realize that we have this power. But this does not mean that we have any ultimate control. "You have no control," said the Voice. "You are as your Soul dictates. You must simply *be,* and your Soul will take care of the rest."

That scared me. What if God loses track of me for a moment? What if my Soul falls asleep on the job? After all that I had suffered, I felt that I deserved some small amount of control, at least enough to make certain that I would never have to endure anything like the pain of my childhood again.

"You are angry, frustrated, and anxious," said the Voice. "You are reaching out for something to keep you in a stable state. I can only respond by telling you to just *be. Be,* without feeling as though you are in control. *Be* with love; *be* with your person; *be* with your Soul, and the powers that matter will act upon you. They will permeate your Soul and foster your *being*. And then you can be without anger, without fear, without frustration and without anxiety.

All of this occurred over many years. It was about four years between the time I learned of the Emotional Body and the time I learned of the Spiritual Body. It was another three years until I learned about the Mental Body, and four more years until I finally learned of the last body: the *Essential Body*.

"There remains a body," said the Voice, "unknown to man, understood by God, to be shared with you in order that you share it with others. It is the Essential Body, the *body of union*. It unites all of the forces of the universe, all of the forces of God, including you, your friends, even your enemies if you have any. It is the body that draws the energies of God into you. It is the place where you may truly connect with others. The Essential Body is your source of wisdom, for it is the energy of all humankind united.

"The Essential Body cannot be fragmented. You may experience it only in its seamless entirety, as a whole, a connection, a relationship. A true relationship, formed in the Essential Body, exists on all levels: physical, emotional, spiritual, and mental. If it does not exist on all of these levels it is not a true relationship. Relationships in the Essential Body are life-long, eternity-long. They interrelate and interconnect, moving you to find another, feel another, reach out to another with your heart's warmth and love, with your mind's thoughts and with your body's feelings.

"The Essential Body represents a seamless, undivided whole, the unity of God, the universe and everything in it. When you enter the world, you are an extension of God, an individual expression of God in its entirety."

CHAPTER 6

Recovery Progresses:
Process and Process Centers

While I was learning about the various bodies, their functions and their significance, I also learned about a treatment modality known as *cranial therapy,* a manual approach to correcting problems of the cranium, as well as the tissues and structures within it. Cranial therapy works by exerting a gentle force on the head and the body. The force decompresses dysfunctional areas and facilitates proper biological rhythms, which in turn provide a foundation for the healthy function of all of the bodies.

These techniques had a profound influence on both my personal and professional lives. I discovered that the key to understanding stress lies in the discharge of repressed emotional energies. This fit nicely with what I had already learned about the Emotional Body, and it resonated with my life experiences. I began to use cranial therapy in an effort to actively open my own Emotional Body. I let go of all of the aspects of my Emotional Body that were manifesting as physical symptoms. I eliminated all the energies that I needed to in order to get on with being—the anger, grief, frustration, depression, fear, and rage. I worked on myself obsessively, using my hands and my mind in tandem. I became adept at the use of imagery and visualization and I read books on self-healing to reinforce the results that I was beginning to see.

All the work paid off beyond my wildest dreams. I gained a new threshold for stress, a greater degree of tolerance, and the ability to live my life in the present without discharging built- up negative energy on my family. I began to make new friends. I taught my colleagues everything that I had learned and they taught me as well. But I still had to face my past: the old hidden traumas; the physical, sexual, and emotional abuse; the events that had scarred me for life. Or had they?

As I continued to learn and to practice, I was finally able to face my past. I released the memories that I had repressed, accepted those who had hurt me and, most importantly, I accepted myself for the person that I am. And as I continued to evolve, so did the people around me—my colleagues, my new friends, my children. Everyone began to find their repressed emotional energies, and they cleared themselves of these obstacles to health and happiness. Each of us cleaned our emotional closets, releasing secrets, memories, forgotten pasts. We developed a new perspective on life (new for most of us, anyway), a positive outlook that had a profound impact on work and family alike.

It was as if we were participating in a new beginning, the emergence of a new world. And as we opened our eyes, our minds, and our hearts, we found that others, only a few at first, but more and more everyday, were participating in the same process. The world around us and the people in it were evolving at an ever-quickening pace, with a clear consciousness that we found beautiful, energizing, and exciting. We rejoiced over the peaceful renaissance of our souls as each of us connected with the *collective unconscious* of our species, our planet, and our universe. We felt blessed and we marveled at the feeling of true wonder for all creation. God loved us. We were God's children.

I became determined to eliminate all evidence of the unhealthy practices of my past. Unfortunately, my husband was unwilling to embark on this journey alongside me. We had been having problems with our relationship, and we agreed upon a divorce. I focused even more attention on my children, and I began to treat them so that they too could release all of the emotional energy that they had repressed during their short lives so that they too could heal. And they flourished as they perceived, understood, and rejoiced alongside me. I became more involved with my children, and for the first time in years I truly experienced the joy of being with them in the present. I surrendered to the purposeful love of my heart and felt myself part of a much larger, completely unified whole.

I looked with renewed vigor at the work of my profession. I saw people every day who suffered through physical and emotional pain. But I had learned that there was no distinction between the two. They are different symptoms of the same underlying problem. I wanted to share more of myself—my knowledge and my experience—in order that more people could learn to foresee, perceive, understand, and rejoice as I had; in order that more people could heal as I had.

I saw the terrible pain, the profound loss of hope and the absolute lack of faith that surrounded me. Together they formed a reflection of the woman I had been. But it was difficult for me to understand those emotions. They were shadows of my past. I felt compelled to work to provide hope to all those that I came in contact with, whether in my professional or my personal life, in order that they too could participate in the new world that I had stepped into. I didn't become a missionary, preaching in an effort to convert others. I taught primarily by example, by *being*.

I dedicated myself increasingly to teaching, traveling all over the country and around the world. I treated addictions, abuses, intolerances, hatreds, and all the other problems that I had worked to remove from my own life. I taught people to uncover their hopes and learn to play. I taught them to teach others. And as people were able to release the emotional energies that afflicted them, I watched faith emerge.

I also continued to learn from the people around me and from the Voice that had helped guide me to this point. The Voice told me about Process, the actualization of the Self through purposeful reflection and discovery. The name Process reflects its dynamic, cyclical nature. Process allows all of the bodies to adjust, realign and communicate with one another. They accept information that fosters communication, which in turn strengthens and enhances their union. They adjust to the new information. They *process* it. They adjust again and they process again. And as all of this occurs, the Self, the integrated alliance of all of the bodies, is able to become clear, present, and focused.

And how does Self initiate Process? What makes the potential of Process a reality? Recall. The bodies *recall* the information that they need.

Process unfolds through the action of *Process Centers*. Each Process Center reaches the Self, the union of all bodies. These centers retain information and they are able to empty that information into the body's tissues so that the Self can communicate about it. They can be divided into *planning centers,* which formulate courses of action, *action centers,* which carry out the plans, and *personal being centers* which facilitate simply being in the present moment, a task considerably more difficult (and important) than it sounds. In order to use these centers to facilitate Recall, the first step is to know where they are located.

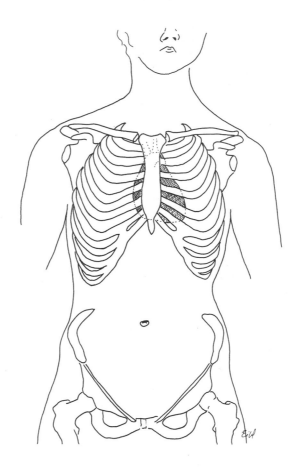

HEART PROCESS CENTER

The most significant Process Center is the heart, which interconnects the spiritual and mental bodies. The heart is the thoroughfare of the Personal Body and the pathway of the Essential Body. It is the key to our awakened state of awareness. The atrioventricular (AV) and sinoatrial (SA) nodes are the home base in the heart for consciousness. Other centers within the heart serve as the home bases for other states and functions.

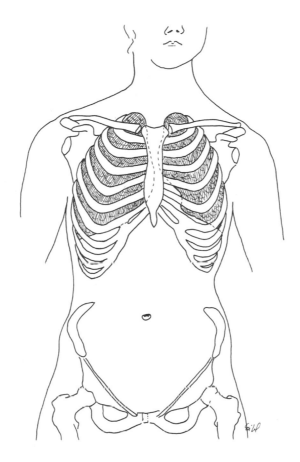

LUNGS PROCESS CENTER

The Process Center of the lungs is also of particular significance for the awakened states. The oxygenation process that the lungs carry out actualizes the incarnation of the Spiritual Body. The lungs are the interface where energies from the universe enter to participate in the Self. As a result the lungs are intimately involved in each individual's daily, soul-directed activities.

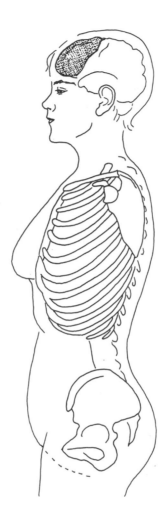

The frontal region (the area of the forehead) is another primary Process Center. This is the Process Center for the Mental Body, for judgment and consideration of the energies in us and around us. The functional practice of the frontal region determines how we respond to those energies.

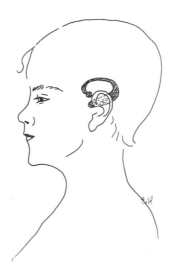

LIMBIC SYSTEM PROCESS CENTER

The limbic system sits inside the core of the brain, but the Process Center is accessed at the bridge of your nose.

The emotion that is significant for this Process Center is rage.

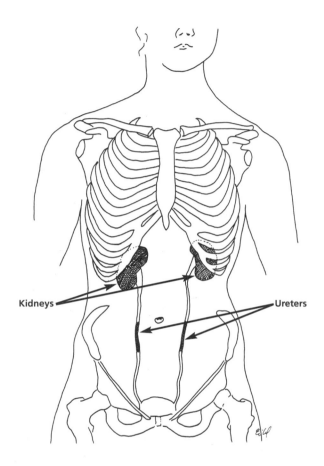

Kidneys   Ureters

KIDNEY AND URETERS PROCESS CENTERS

The kidneys are the Process Center responsible for handling fear. Fear may underlie any emotional state, including, but not limited to, anger, frustration, and depression. Fear resides in the kidneys, including fear of life and fear of God.

The ureters are a Process Center that promotes drainage of all toxins. This Process Center can be used as a powerful first-aid tool.

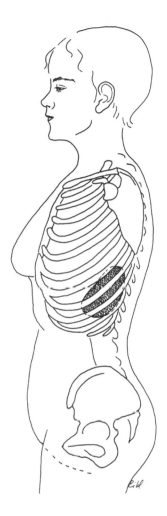

SPLEEN PROCESS CENTER

The spleen is the seat of disappointment in humankind. If this disappointment becomes too strong, it can replace the service that is originally programmed into the Essential Body—service to humankind in the name of God.

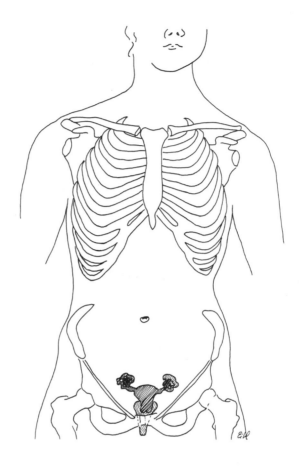

SEXUAL ORGANS PROCESS CENTER

Our sexual organs also act as a Process Center. It is within this Process Center that who we are in this life becomes clear.

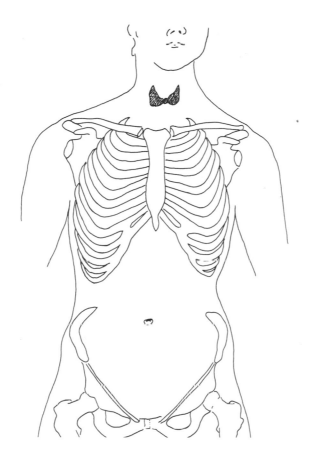

THYROID PROCESS CENTER

The thyroid is the Process Center responsible for interrelations, affecting the interface of humans with each other as well as the interface of humans and the universe. In doing so, it carries out a primary function of the Essential Body.

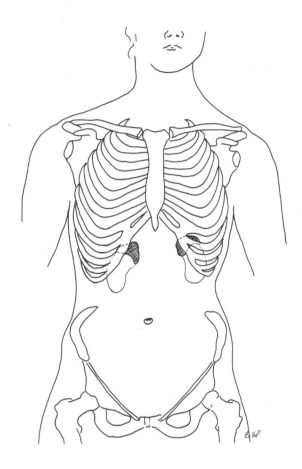

Stress thresholds are regulated in the adrenals.

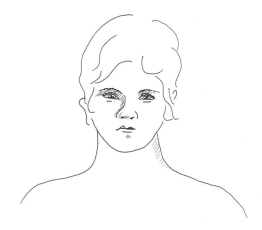

EYES PROCESS CENTER

Our eyes can discover who we are, what we are and what we may become. This Process Center is the fountain of the spiritual, emotional, personal, and essential bodies.

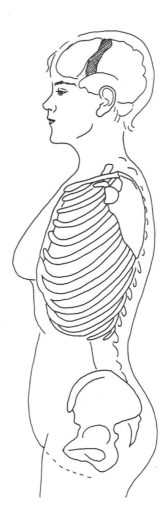

PARIETAL LOBES PROCESS CENTER

The parietal lobes (also referred to as the *motor cortex*) represent the site of action. This Process Center orients our bodies in the direction of our own individual journey.

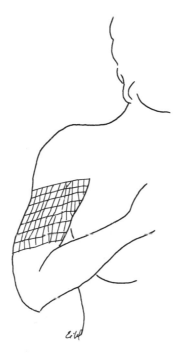

UPPER ARMS PROCESS CENTER

The upper arms are our *self-control centers*. They represent our destiny in the present, as well as our means of transcending it.

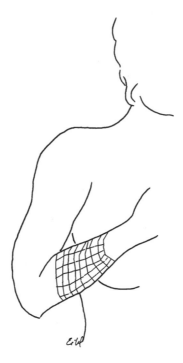

The forearms are the seat of our belief systems. Whether we are rigid or relaxed in this center will determine whether our beliefs will facilitate the alliance of our bodies or work to keep this alliance from guiding our journey.

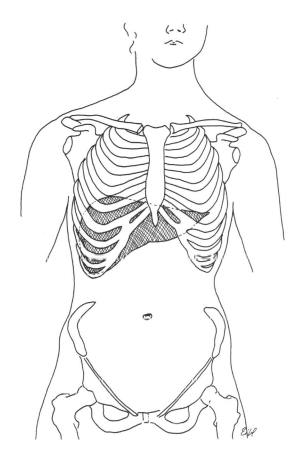

LIVER PROCESS CENTER

The liver is the secondary Process Center where the bodies detoxify. It facilitates the elimination of physical body toxins, Emotional Body toxins, Spiritual Body toxins, Mental Body toxins, and Personal Body toxins.

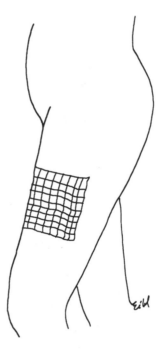

UPPER THIGHS PROCESS CENTER

The upper thighs are our activity Process Centers. They can help us to travel smoothly through life, or they can cause us to become entrenched in the past and the future, at the expense of the present. Using these Process Centers, we can achieve a momentum in the present that allows us to be and do simultaneously.

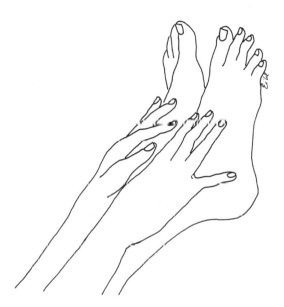

HANDS AND FEET PROCESS CENTER

The hands and feet are our tools for being. The Process Centers here are programmed with our plan of action for this life.

A SUMMARY OF PROCESS CENTERS

PROCESS CENTER	SIGNIFICANCE
Heart	Interconnects the spiritual and mental bodies Awareness and consciousness
Lungs	Oxygenation Daily, soul-directed activities
Frontal Region	Judgement, cognition Mental Body
Limbic System	Rage Survival
Kidney	Fear
Ureters	Drainage of toxins First-aid
Spleen	Disappointment in humankind
Sexual Organs	Who we are in life
Thyroid	Interrelations How we interface with the universe
Adrenals	Stress thresholds
Eyes	Who we are What we are What we may become
Parietal Lobes	Action Direction of individual journey
Upper Arms	Self-control
Forearms	Belief systems
Liver	Detoxification
Upper Thighs	Activity
Hands and Feet	Tools for being Plan of action for this life

Recall

In this second part, I introduce Neurofascial Process as a technique that can help you recall emotional pain to help you heal wounds. Often our wounds—particularly emotional wounds—have been covered over for many years, during which remarkable growth has occurred in spite of them. Our emotions can be repressed in our bodies within the physical tissues. What are our emotions? Joy, fear, happiness, sorrow, anger—these are our most important emotions. They are our natural responses to what happens in our lives, but many people repress strong emotional energies, and it is the view of most professionals in the field of psychotherapeutics that is the way to emotional dis-ease. I and many other mind-body professionals believe that emotional energies repressed in the body often result in pain and suffering. Yet that does *not* mean "it is all in your head." Indeed, pain is in the body. It is perceived in the brain, and often projected through the body tissues. Why then look at repressed emotional energies? Sometimes, those energies block tissues and cause a great deal of pain and disability.

Emotions are within us. I generate my own emotions just as I generate my own thoughts. Both are driven by energies. Many believe in the great psychologist Carl Jung's concept of the "collective unconscious." Jung claimed that our thoughts exist before we think them in an unconscious world that we all share. But whether or not this is true, once *you* think the thought, you now *own* that thought. It is inside you, it is part of you. Part II of this deals with emotional energies, thought energies, and other disturbances inside you which, when repressed, are experienced as pain in your body.

I did not begin my own self-healing and my work with healing others by looking for repressed emotions. I was looking for ways to treat pain, disease, and disability. At first I was satisfied, but eventually this was not enough. I wanted to get rid of *all* of my pain. I wanted to heal all my children's ailments: cognitive, respiratory, cardiac, learning, behavioral. This drove me to look beneath the superficial problems. I found that these problems were a veritable Pandora's Box.

What is the real story of Pandora's Box? Pandora opened up the box and many unpleasant things leapt out of it; but when she got to the bottom of the box, she found treasure. What was the treasure at the bottom of Pandora's box? Hope! What if Pandora had never opened the box? What if she had never looked inside and allowed all those *other* things to come out of her box? She would never have discovered hope. What a pity that would have been.

Your own body and its repressed emotions and energies are *your* Pandora's Box; and Recall and Neurofascial Process are the easiest, safest means to open it, so that you can discover the hope that waits within.

CHAPTER 7

Process Centers

Once we have located the Process Centers, as presented in Part I, we must connect them to our organs in order to facilitate the dual activities of *Recall* and *Process*. This is done by placing hands (your own, a friend's, a family member's, or a therapist's) on the various Process Centers as described in the following pages. The pictures will help you to achieve the proper positions. Place your hands softly, without fear. You will feel your "bodies" shifting, changing, letting go. They may begin to move of their own volition. You may see, hear or feel new sensations, and if you follow the instructions, positive changes will be evident.

Perform the exercises in a peaceful, relaxing environment. You may choose to leave the light on or off, although darkness can help to facilitate the deep state of relaxation that you will experience. You may practice sitting up or lying down—whichever is most appealing to you. Leave your hands in each position for at least fifteen minutes at a time. If you feel anything at all—a tingle, a movement, an easier breathing pattern—anything—then continue with that position for half an hour. If, after half an hour, it still feels as though something is happening to your body—if tissues are shifting or even if you feel as though you are relaxing—then hold the position for up to an hour. You may go through all the positions and then return to any one of them where it felt like some change was happening.

Recall will bring long-repressed emotional energy to the surface in a nonthreatening manner, so you should be prepared to deal with, or process, these emotions. Once you begin, pay careful attention to everything that you feel during and after each exercise, no matter how vague or insignificant it may seem. Remember, nothing is trivial. You may notice positive changes in your stress levels, your fears and your movement. You may find yourself becoming increasingly serene, patient, and tolerant of those around you. You may find your life easier, more pleasant. By practicing Recall, you may find a new aspect of yourself that will talk to you, be with you, guide you into a new world. As you perform these exercises, listen for the voice of your soul, and put your faith in it.

CHAPTER 8

The Heart:
Beginning Process

B ecause the heart is the most important Process Center, it is the best place to start. You should ask yourself if you have any heart traumas. These usually involve the love, or lack thereof, between you and a parent, sibling, spouse, friend, lover, or anyone else close to you. Ask yourself if you are able to love. Ask yourself if you want to continue along on autopilot, with nothing but your mind to guide you, or if perhaps it would be a happier journey if your heart were able to interface with both your mind and your soul. Wouldn't it be nice to travel through life with a direct connection to your Spiritual Body? These heart exercises will enable you to rejoin life with a rejuvenated heart that will be able to process your bodies' energies in a manner that will allow you to express your own unique personality traits.

Hold each position for at least fifteen minutes before going on to the next. Hold it longer if you feel something happening, or else return to it after you have gone through all the positions.

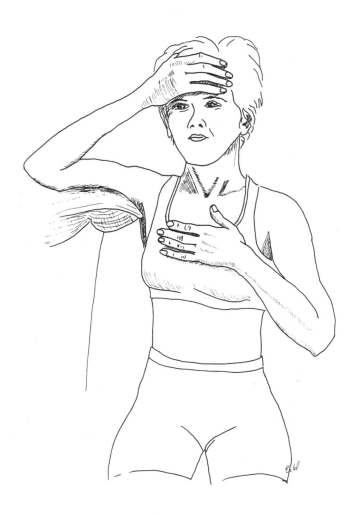

HEART AND FOREHEAD

- Begin by placing one hand on your heart and the other on your forehead, or frontal region. This may trigger a change in judgment or a shift in your worldview.

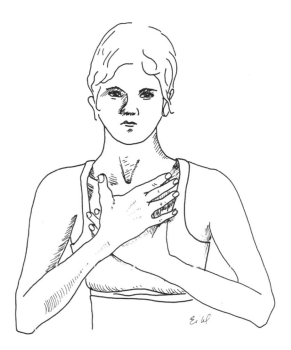

HEART AND LUNGS

- Next place one hand on your heart and the other on your lungs. You may notice a shift in your breathing.

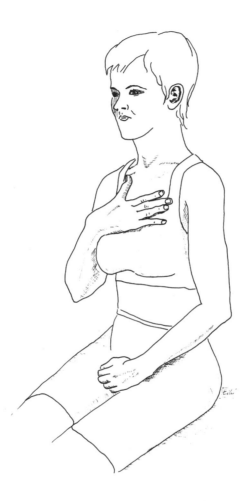

HEART AND SEXUAL ORGANS

• Place one hand on your heart and the other on your sexual organs. You may experience enjoyable sensations during this exercise.

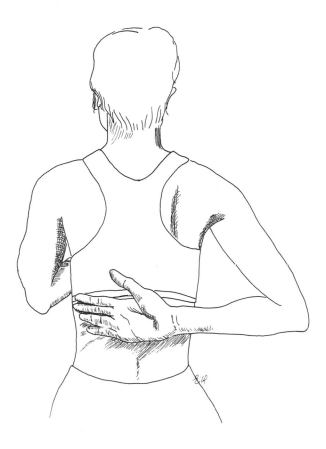

HEART AND KIDNEYS

• Place one hand on your heart and the other on your kidneys. Your fears should begin to subside.

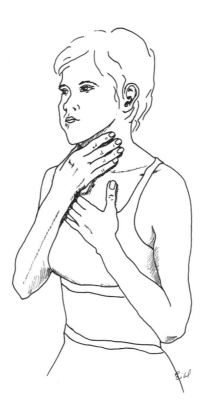

- Next place a hand on your heart and place the other on your thyroid gland.

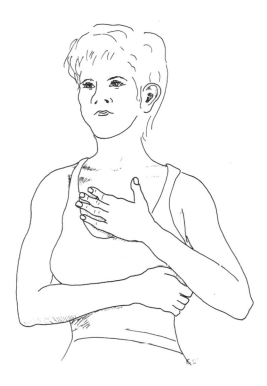

HEART AND SPLEEN

• Place a hand on your heart and a hand on your spleen.

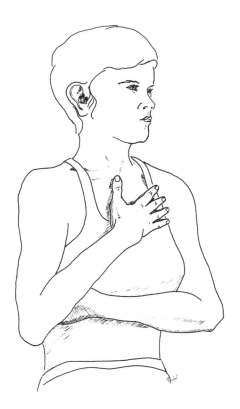

HEART AND LIVER

- Place one hand on your heart and the other on your liver. Anger is stored in the liver, so be prepared for the release of anger energy.

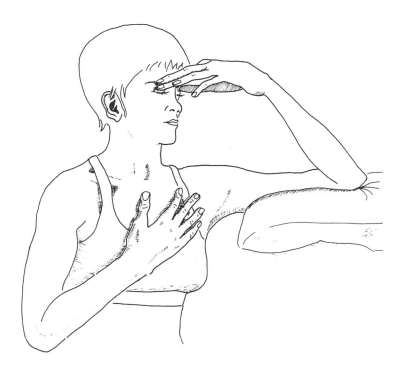

HEART AND EYES

• Finally, place one hand on your heart and the other on your eyes.
  We generally see only what our conscious mind allows us to see,
  but this exercise can open up other types of vision.

CHAPTER 9

The Limbic System

N ext you will be working with your limbic system, a portion of the brain buried deep within your cerebral cortex. The limbic system is much older, from an evolutionary perspective, than the cortex itself (the outermost part of the brain), which we have in common with all mammals. It is an automatic driving force during periods of decreased self-control. When you are frightened, severely stressed, or weakened due to illness or injury, your limbic system will respond.

The limbic system is also associated with rage. A direct blow to the head can affect the limbic system, causing an individual to become more aggressive. This new behavior cannot be consciously controlled. It is the limbic system's response to the dangers associated with a traumatic head injury. If an individual is prone to outbursts of rage, loses control of his or her emotions (often for no apparent reason), or cannot be in an excessively stimulating environment without becoming aggressive, that individual may have a damaged or overstimulated limbic system.

This type of injury to the limbic system is more common than most people realize. Many of us banged our heads growing up, and often the incidents are forgotten and the results of the injury ignored. But the response of the limbic system is evident to a trained observer, and can also be visible to the untrained eye.

Stand in front of a mirror and observe your own frontonasal area (around the bridge of your nose). Often there is an indentation of the forehead over the nose, or a sharp recession at the frontonasal site, indicating that trauma may have affected the limbic system. If this area is smooth, there may still be excessive stimulation of the limbic system. The following techniques can help to relax or repair the limbic system, eliminating the symptoms caused by its dysfunction.

Hold each position for at least fifteen minutes before proceeding.

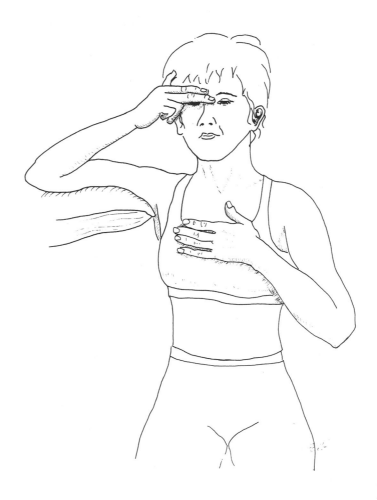

LIMBIC SYSTEM AND HEART

- Place one hand on the bridge of your nose and the other on your
  heart.

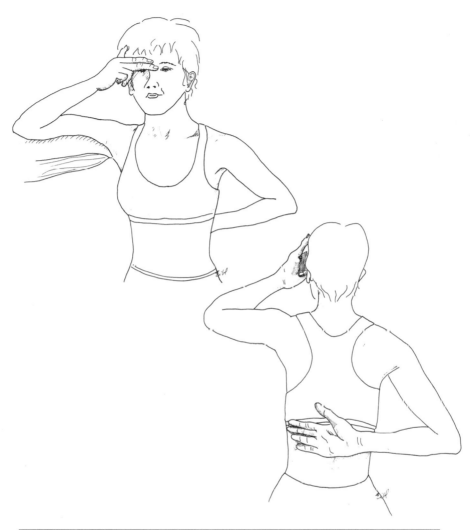

LIMBIC SYSTEM AND KIDNEYS

• Place one hand on the bridge of your nose and the other on your kidneys.

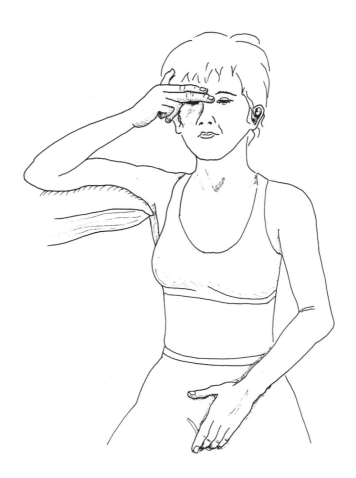

LIMBIC SYSTEM AND SEXUAL ORGANS

- Place one hand on the bridge of your nose and the other on your sexual organs.

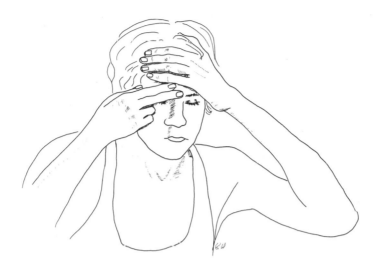

LIMBIC SYSTEM AND FOREHEAD

- Place one hand on the bridge of your nose and the other on your forehead.

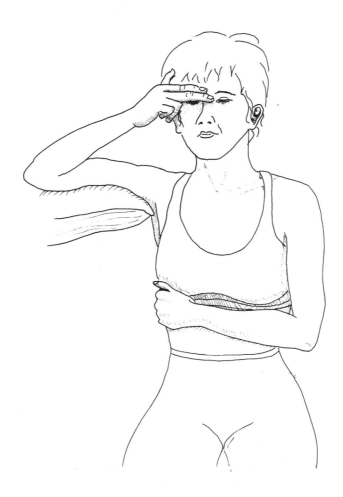

LIMBIC SYSTEM AND LIVER

- Place one hand on the bridge of your nose and the other on your liver.

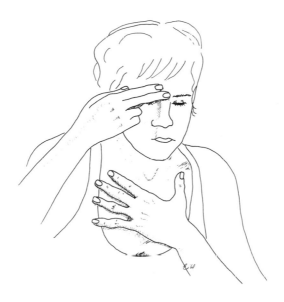

LIMBIC SYSTEM AND LUNGS

- Place one hand on the bridge of your nose and the other on your lungs. Spread the hand as wide as possible, in order to cover the maximum possible amount of your lungs.

CHAPTER 10

The Kidneys

I touched on the prevalence of fear earlier, and mentioned that the kidneys are the seat of fear. Many people accept fear as a normal part of their lives. There are things it is natural and healthy to be afraid of. For example, fear of jumping off of a 500-foot cliff or fear of stepping in front of a speeding car are both survival expedients which generally help us more than they hinder us. But fear is also one of the primary reasons that many lives lack momentum and direction. People may be immobilized by their fears; they may be unable to act, speak, or even think freely for fear that something horrible will happen to them. They may even be afraid of their feelings. This fear of feelings usually stems from our inability to understand them.

Fear is generally not a desirable consort. It can isolate us, inhibit our activities, and drain us of our energy. As you perform the following exercises, which all involve the kidneys, focus on your fear. Confront it as it surfaces, and you will marvel at the changes in yourself. Once again, hold each position for fifteen minutes, giving more time to positions that produce an inner reaction.

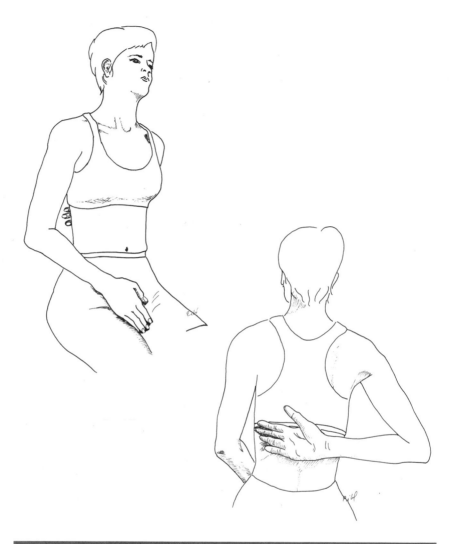

KIDNEYS AND SEXUAL ORGANS

• Place one hand on your kidneys and the other on your sexual organs.

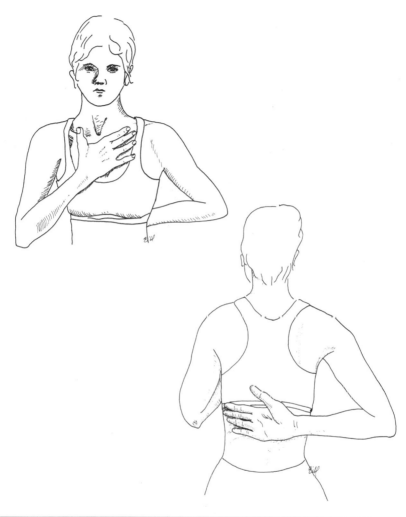

KIDNEYS AND LUNGS

• Place one hand on your kidneys and the other on your lungs.

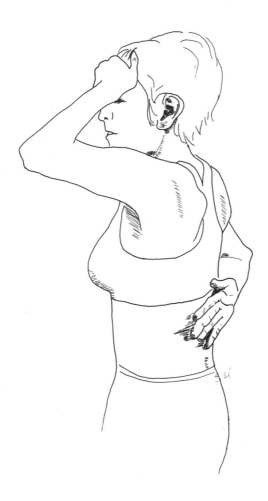

KIDNEYS AND FOREHEAD

- Place one hand on your kidneys and the other on the frontal region (forehead).

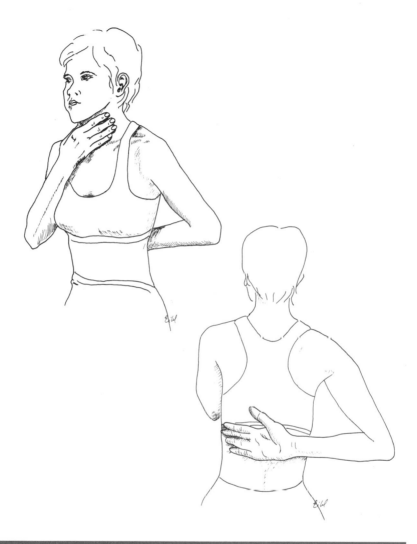

KIDNEYS AND THYROID

- Place one hand on your kidneys and the other hand over the thyroid gland at the front of the lower neck.

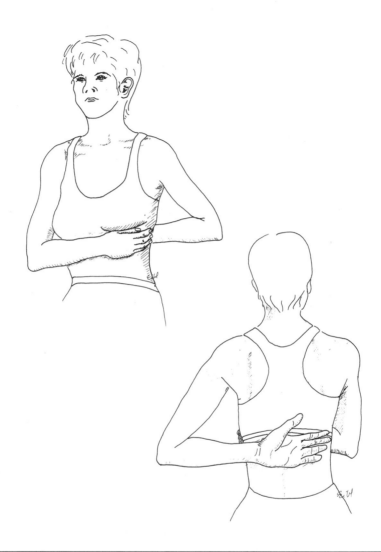

KIDNEYS AND SPLEEN

• Place one hand on your kidneys and the other on your spleen.

CHAPTER 11

The Frontal Region

For some people, learning does not come easily. They study and study, but cannot absorb the material. They hear when they are spoken to, but they cannot process and integrate the information. Perhaps their judgment is inappropriate, their attention span is short, or concentration is difficult. All of these symptoms indicate dysfunction in the frontal region, which is the seat of planning, judgment, attention, and concentration. Frontal process problems are common in both children and adults. These problems can be caused by illness or injury. By treating the frontal region, many symptoms can be eliminated. Again, hold each position for at least fifteen minutes, before going on to the next. Hold it longer if you feel something happening, or else return to it after you have gone through all the positions.

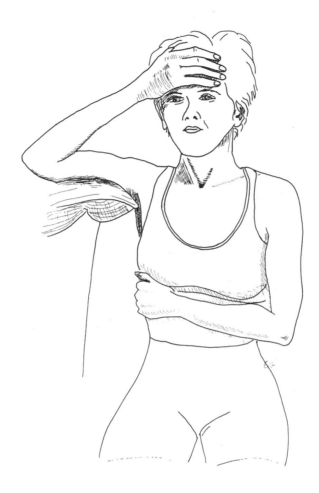

FRONTAL REGION AND LIVER

• Place one hand on your forehead and the other hand on your liver.

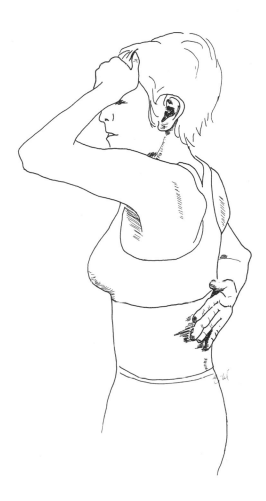

FRONTAL REGION AND KIDNEYS

• Place one hand on your forehead and the other on your kidneys.

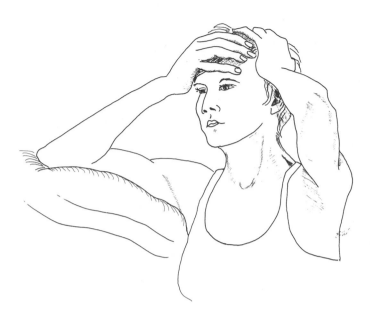

FRONTAL REGION AND LEFT PARIETAL

- Place one hand on your forehead, and the other on the left parietal region. Then repeat this replacing the left parietal region with the same area on the right hand side.

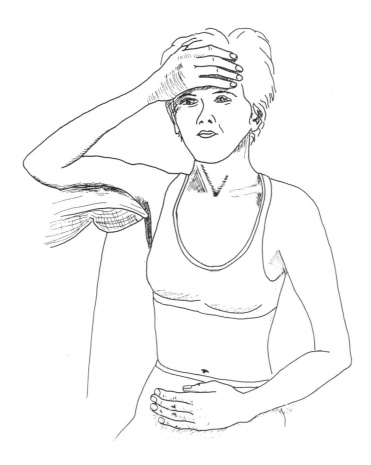

FRONTAL REGION AND ABDOMEN

• Place one hand on your forehead and the other hand on your lower abdomen. This will affect the digestive system.

Working with the Process Center in the frontal region can help us with more issues than those associated with planning, concentration, and judgment. For instance, many people do not appreciate their physical body. We want to feel beautiful when we look in the mirror, but our society's narrow definition of beauty makes it difficult, if not impossible to do so. To complicate things further, each of us tends to be our own toughest critic. Even when others find us attractive, sometimes we are unable to observe any evidence either of our internal or external beauty.

Pressures regarding the physical body are very real. This has increased the prevalence of many illnesses, including eating disorders like anorexia, bulimia, and morbid obesity. Many of these problems stem from personal issues that we have not addressed. Thoughts and feelings may take the form of energy that can adversely affect the physical body. We feel stressed, unhappy or isolated, but because we have repressed the feelings that are causing the problems, we are unable to understand why we feel as we do. Treating the Process Center in the frontal region can help us to identify and eliminate the causes of these problems. Hold the following positions as in other exercises.

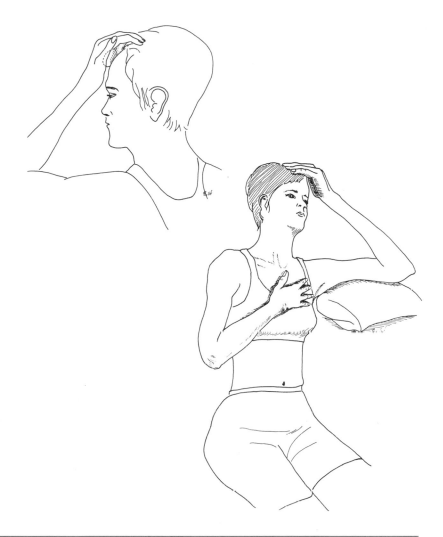

FRONTAL REGION AND HEART

• Place a hand one inch above the left side of the forehead, so that it is not actually making contact with your body. Place your other hand on your heart.

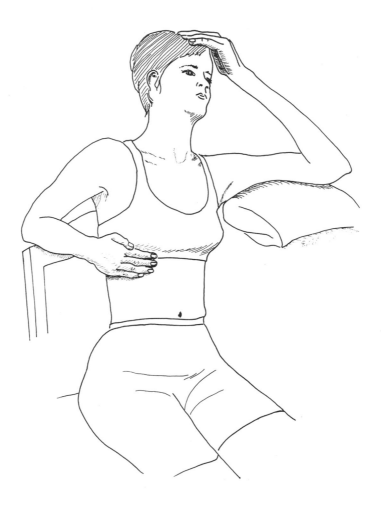

FRONTAL REGION AND LIVER

- Next place one hand one inch above the left side of the forehead, so that it is not actually touching it. Place your other hand over your liver.

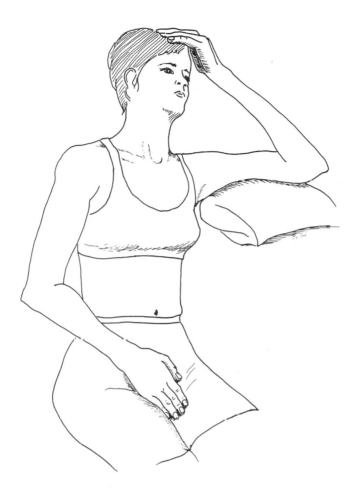

- Place one hand one inch above the left side of the forehead, so that it is not actually touching it. Place your other hand on your sexual organs.

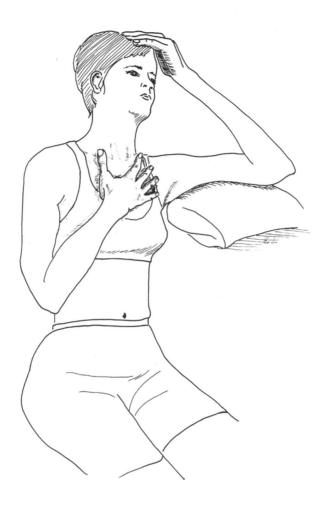

FRONTAL REGION AND LUNGS

- Place one hand one inch above the left side of the forehead, so that it does not touch it. Spread the other hand over your chest, covering as much of your lungs as you possibly can.

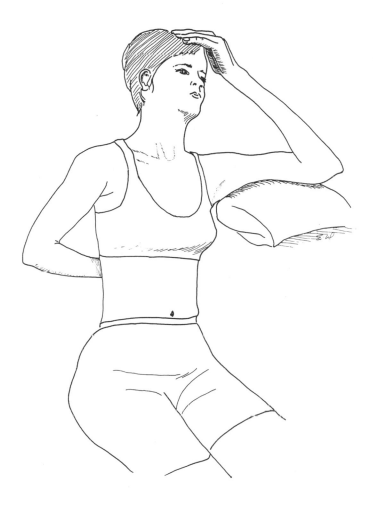

FRONTAL REGION AND KIDNEYS

- Place one hand one inch above the left side of the forehead, not touching it, and put the other hand on your kidneys.

CHAPTER 12

The Lungs

When we are born, our first breath is a new beginning. It represents our entry into this world, and it is our first awareness of our life and our bodies. We literally come alive. But as life goes on, we may begin to feel disconnected from our bodies. The awareness that we gained with that first breath is suppressed, or lost. Often we are not even aware that part of us is not functioning properly. In other cases we may feel a vague numbness. It may seem as though there is a lack of life in some part of us, but we cannot discern what has changed. Through work with the lungs, this problem can be corrected. Hold each position for at least fifteen minutes before going on to the next. Hold it longer if you feel something happening, or else return to it after you have gone through all the positions.

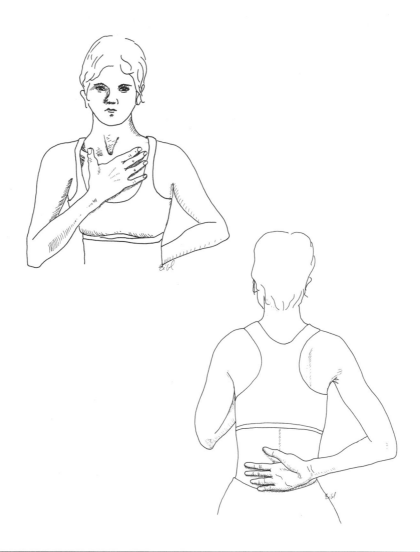

LUNGS AND URETERS

- Place one hand across your chest, spreading your fingers wide in order to cover as much of your lungs as possible. Place your other hand in the small of your back.

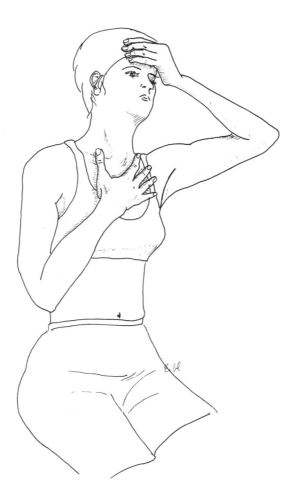

LUNGS AND FOREHEAD

- Place one hand across your chest, spreading your fingers wide in order to cover as much of your lungs as possible. Place your other hand on your forehead.

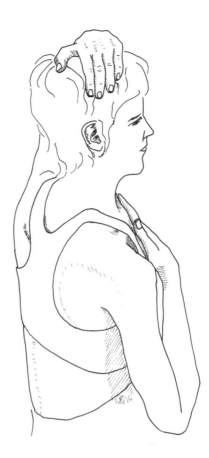

LUNGS AND PARIETALS

- Place one hand across your chest, spreading your fingers wide in order to cover as much of your lungs as possible. Place your other hand on the crown of your head.

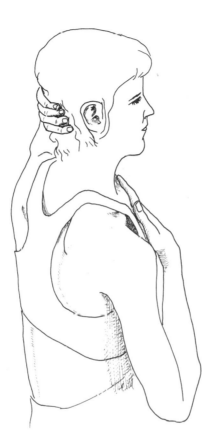

LUNGS AND BRAINSTEM

- Place one hand across your chest, spreading your fingers wide in order to cover as much of your lungs as possible. Place the other hand on the back of your head just above the top of your neck.

CHAPTER 13

Conclusion

These are the wonders of the universe, the wonders of the soul, the wonders of God. When we begin to recognize the physical, emotional, spiritual, mental, personal and essential bodies, we can use them to heal. And they can allow us to live a more meaningful existence.

Before I began the process of Recall, I felt incomplete. I had worldly success, wonderful children, and many friends, but I was never truly content. The pain of my past haunted me. It chased me through life nipping at my heels like a rabid dog. I feared that it would lunge for my throat if I let my guard down or turned to face it. Recall allowed me to tame the beast that was my past. I made it a part of my Self so that it couldn't cause me any more pain.

Each of us has suffered in our own way. We have formed memories and repressed those memories. And we have sworn to ourselves, consciously or unconsciously, that one day we would awaken to the present and discover the promise of life. Now is the time to awaken. There is a readiness now far beyond that of previous generations to learn the difference between hiding from the past, living in the future, and being in the present. We can recall, and in doing so we can initiate the process of aligning our various bodies so that they can communicate in a meaningful fashion. We can recover; we can heal the wounds of the past and focus on the joy and love of the present. Don't be bashful. Accept yourself for who you are: you are God. Take your life in your own two hands, literally and figuratively, and begin the process that will make you complete. *Recall.*

PART III

Protocols for
Neurofascial Process

W hat is Neurofascial Process? It is an approach to self-healing. The exercises in Part II were in fact the Neurofascial Processes for the treatment of emotional-based traumas, mental stress, and other endogenous forms of dysfunction. But perhaps you are not at the present time particularly interested in looking at the emotional traumas of the past. Part III offers Neurofascial Processes for dealing with pain and physical problems that exist in the present. When Neurofascial Process first emerged in the early 1980s, it was for the purpose of treating physical ailments. A most remarkable treatment approach, it can be used for all pain and physical dysfunction, no matter how chronic or how severe.

I have included simple anatomical diagrams to help you visualize the region of your problem. Each technique or group of techniques has its own anatomical drawing of the region to which it is to be applied. There are also photographs of each region. Place *your* hands in the positions on the body just as the hands are placed in the photograph.

You can use any or all of the treatment techniques in Part III for any region of the body. Even if you have never experienced any pain or discomfort in that region, you may still discover that there is room for improvement: increased ease of movement, more movement throughout the region, greater strength and increased endurance. Perhaps you are not aware of any knee problems, yet perhaps you would enjoy going for walks and would like to walk faster. Perhaps you would like to try running, but are afraid you would not have the stamina. Treat your knee, hip and ankle with *all* of the protocols outlined in the ankle, knee, and hip sub-sections. Then test your strength, function, and endurance. You may be quite surprised. Perhaps you can run in spite of your age, your history, or your beliefs about yourself.

This section of the book contains many *protocols*. What is a protocol? A protocol is like a formula. It is an orderly set of steps for you to follow. Each protocol addresses discomfort such as low back pain or knee pain, and other issues such as learning disabilities or stress.

We all can perform all of these Neurofascial Process techniques. You can use any of them at any time. You can perform one a day. You can perform several each day. You will not usually lose whatever gains you make with the techniques you perform. This means: if you perform a technique today for thirty minutes and you feel relief, relief will not go away. Whatever changes have occurred will probably still be present in another week, month, or year.

Neurofascial Process requires both hands. Each hand is placed on a separate region of the body. Usually one hand is on a Process Center. The Process Centers are universal. What does that mean? Every person alive uses these same areas for processing energies. We all use the same Process Centers for the same energies.

You can perform most protocols without assistance. Usually Neurofascial Process is quite simple. Place one hand on one location as indicated in the protocol and in the illustration. Place the second hand on the other location. For some regions it may be a bit more difficult to reach the indicated spot. For example, it may be difficult to reach behind your back high enough to contact the kidneys, especially if you have a shoulder joint problem. Certainly it is impossible to put your hand on the back of your lungs. But each Process Center is unique and important. There is no substitute. If you have to reach the back of the lungs as a Process Center, you will have to seek help, perhaps the hands of a friend or family member.

Neurofascial Process can be performed for as long as you want. You can have a one-hour session. You can have a five-hour session. There are no precautions or contraindications regarding performing the exercises for too long a time. On the other hand, a Neurofascial Process session *can* be too brief. A session should not be less than twenty minutes. If you only have ten minutes, you are possibly wasting your time.

If you want to perform several techniques simultaneously, obtain the assistance of friends or family—there are no precautions or contraindications. Simply have your helpers' hands placed on your body at the appropriate locations. For example, you can use six hands with three people. One hand of each helper will be on the Process Centers; then have them place their other hands on the other locations indicated by the protocol. A lot of healing can take place at one session with three or more persons involved. You might even have a Neurofascial Process party where you take turns being the subject of the session.

If you have a very ill person in your home, or are concerned about someone in the hospital or in a nursing home, why not invite his or her family or friends to perform a many-handed Neurofascial Process? The more the work is performed, the faster you will see results.

What more is there to say about Neurofascial Process? You really can use this approach for any pain, disorder, disease, or disability. You do not have to limit yourself to the locations named in this book. For example, if you hurt your nose, place one hand on your nose, then the second hand on the ureters, for first aid. Continue with Neurofascial Process between your nose and your heart. Continue afterwards with other Process Centers, until you have performed Neurofascial Process from your nose to all of the Process Centers outlined in Part II and III of this book.

You are not limited in how many total hours you perform Neurofascial Process. Essentially you can and should continue for as long as it takes for healing to be complete. You can stop at any time. You can start or restart at any time. There are no limitations to the outcomes with this work. Give yourself a chance. Treat your children, your spouse, your mother and father and sister and brother. Give this book to a friend. Keep it by the bed so that you remember to perform some Neurofascial Process before you go to bed and when you get up in the morning.

You can progress slowly. You can go as fast as you wish. The more Neurofascial Process you perform, the quicker you will heal. You can do this self-healing one day a week, or one day a month. You can do this treatment every day for the rest of your life. You can choose to heal quickly.

Review the protocols as listed on the contents pages of this book. The protocols are listed alphabetically. The word "pain" is present in the titles for most of them. This means: the technique works well whenever there is pain. Choose the bodily regions or organs where you are ailing, and practice the protocols.

How does Neurofascial Process, work? We don't really know, but here is my hypothesis: there is a closing of internal "circuitry"—a connection made between the body parts when two hands touch different areas. It is as if the body parts are "discussing" the problem within. Your hands are only facilitating the connection.

The rest of this book contains the protocols. Enjoy!

ABDOMEN
Stomachache; Gastritis; Ulcers; Irritable Bowel Syndrome; Diverticulitis; Ileitis

We live at a time in which abdominal ailments of many varieties are very common. Our food and water are often polluted by microbes that cause abdominal infections. Antibiotics are becoming less and less effective against them, due to the evolution of strains of microbes that are resistant to their power. (The danger of these resistant strains is well described in *The Coming Plague* by Laurie Garrett.) Just popping a pill to cure our illness is no longer a viable option. But even when they are effective against infection, antibiotics can negatively affect your stomach, your intestines, and your bowel. If you are suffering from chronic or acute abdominal problems, Neurofascial process may provide an appropriate alternative.

Pain or problems in the abdomen may stem from any of the organs and functions of the gastrointestinal tract, including: the cardiac sphincter (where the esophagus and stomach join); the duodenum, especially the first and second portions of the duodenum; the small intestines (on the right side of the ileum and the left side of the jejunum); the

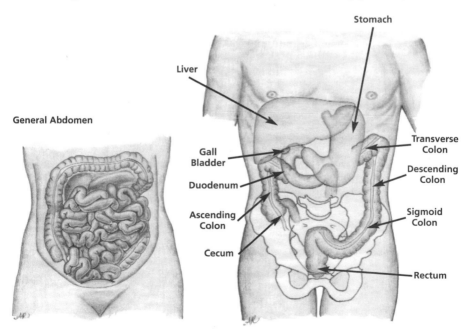

General Abdomen

Stomach

Liver

Gall Bladder

Duodenum

Ascending Colon

Cecum

Transverse Colon

Descending Colon

Sigmoid Colon

Rectum

ileocecal valve (where the ileum joins the cecum); the sigmoid colon (the source of irritable bowel syndrome and diverticulitis); the large intestine, including the ascending colon, the place of colitis, ulcerative colitis, and Crohn's disease; the liver; the gall bladder.

It is possible to treat the organs of the abdomen as a whole, by placing your hand over the general area of the abdomen where you are experiencing the problem. It is also possible to treat them individually, if you are aware of which organ or organs are the source of the difficulty. It may be helpful to acquire an anatomy atlas and look up each of the above organs in turn, so that you can become familiar with their precise positions in your body.

STEP 1

Consider first whatever general area is in pain. If there is infection, bloating and pain of unknown origin, or whether the problem is acute or chronic, try the ureters as a Process Center.

- Place one hand behind the low back, on the ureters.
- Place the second hand over the abdomen. Explore each of the following organs, either together or one at a time: stomach, cardiac sphincter, duodenum, small intestines, ileocecal valve, large intestines, sigmoid colon, liver, gall bladder. If you have family or friends who can participate, you can contact as many organs at a time as your wish.

Do not limit your time. Hold each of these hand placements for at least one hour. If there is the least amount of change, for example tenderness over the region, or more motion in the surrounding tissues, continue. When there is a significant *leaky gut syndrome* (means that the wall of the organ has excessive permeability) treatment should continue for up to twenty hours. During treatment, you will experience continuing changes in the amount of pain, pressure, bloating, digestion, etc.

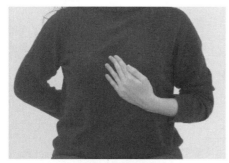

URETERS AND CARDIAC SPHINCTER

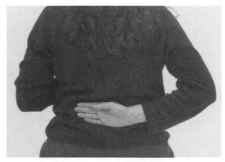

URETERS AND CARDIAC SPHINCTER (REAR VIEW)

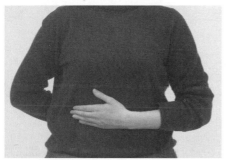

URETERS AND DUODENUM

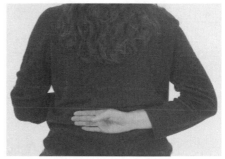

URETERS AND DUODENUM (REAR VIEW)

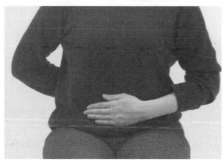

URETERS AND SMALL INTESTINE

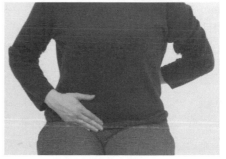

URETERS AND ILEOCECAL VALVE

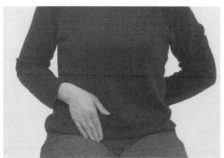

URETERS AND ASCENDING COLON

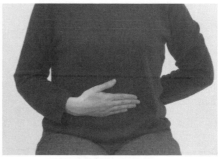

URETERS AND TRANSVERSE COLON

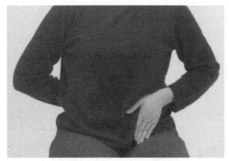

URETERS AND DESCENDING COLON

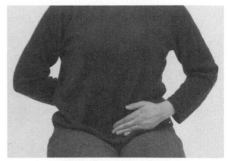

URETERS AND SIGMOID COLON

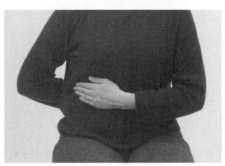

URETERS AND LIVER

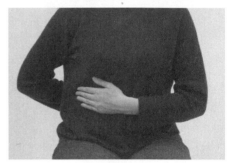

URETERS AND GALL BLADDER

STEP 2

It is always beneficial to follow the initial phase of healing work for the gastrointestinal tract by performing Neurofascial Process to the kidneys. Both kidneys, as well as the liver, utilize complex methods for the excretion of toxins. Many toxins will be excreted via the kidneys. Once the ureters are open with Step 2, it is useful to connect hand placements between the following organs with the kidneys: stomach, cardiac sphincter, duodenum, small intestines, ileocecal valve, large intestines, sigmoid colon, liver, gall bladder.

- Place one hand behind the back, over the bottom rib, on the kidneys.

- Place the second hand hand on the following organs in turn: stomach, cardiac sphincter, duodenum, small intestines, ileocecal valve, large intestines, sigmoid colon, liver, gall bladder. If you have family or friends who can participate, you can contact as many organs at a time as you wish.

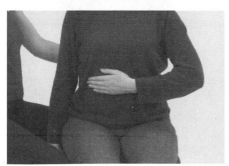

KIDNEYS AND CARDIAC SPHINCTER

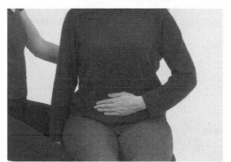

KIDNEYS AND CARDIAC SPHINCTER (REAR VIEW)

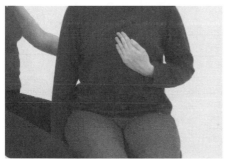

KIDNEYS AND DUODENUM

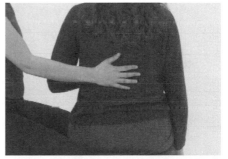

KIDNEYS AND SMALL INTESTINE

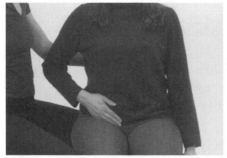

KIDNEYS AND ILEOCECAL VALVE

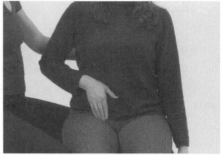

KIDNEYS AND ASCENDING COLON

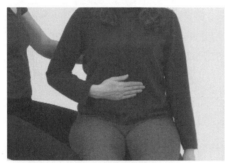

KIDNEYS AND TRANSVERSE COLON

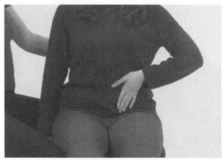

KIDNEYS AND DESCENDING COLON

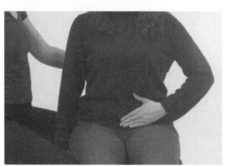

KIDNEYS AND SIGMOID COLON

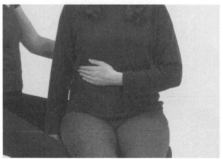

KIDNEYS AND LIVER

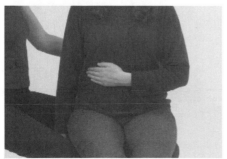

KIDNEYS AND GALL BLADDER

STEP 3

As mentioned above in Step 2, the kidneys and the liver are major excretion routes for toxins. The liver is responsible for determining which matter will be sent to cells as metabolites for nutrients, and which is toxic matter and will be sent for excretion.

- Place one hand over the liver.
- Place the second hand on all of the following organs either all together or one at a time: stomach, cardiac sphincter, duodenum, small intestines, ileocecal valve, large intestines, sigmoid colon, liver, gall bladder. If you have family or friends who can participate, you can contact as many organs at a time as you wish.

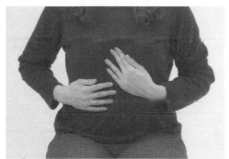

LIVER AND CARDIAC SPHINCTER

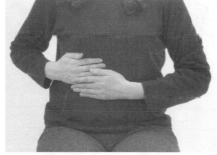

LIVER AND DUODENUM

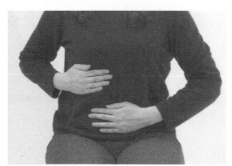

LIVER AND SMALL INTESTINE

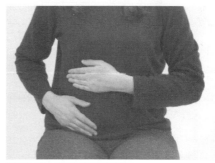

LIVER AND ILEOCECAL VALVE

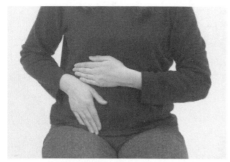

LIVER AND ASCENDING COLON

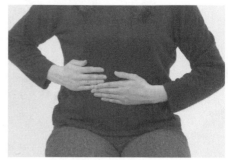

LIVER AND TRANSVERSE COLON

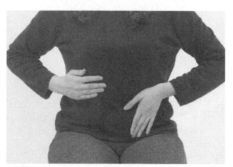

LIVER AND DESCENDING COLON

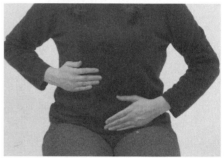

LIVER AND SIGMOID COLON

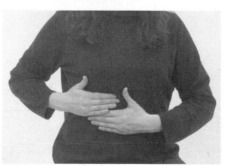

LIVER AND GALL BLADDER

Maintain the hand placements for as long as you feel symptoms and signs are subsiding. Perhaps by this time you are digesting better; perhaps your bowels are moving better; perhaps you are less bloated; perhaps you are eating better.

Continue for as long as you wish. There are no precautions or contraindications.

STEP 4

Many emotions, thoughts, and perceptions are associated with food, eating, digestion, and excretion. Eating disorders are common. The physical and emotional aspects of such problems are usually interrelated. Sometimes it is impossible to tell which came first: Was the person first anorexic, unable to force food into their mouth? Or was there first a physical component, a restriction that compromised digestion and excretion? Is there a history of suppositories, colonics, constipation, or diarrhea? Are shame and self-consciousness or humiliation and embarrassment part of the history? Due to years of medications are you convinced that you will never be able to eat again without consequences of heartburn, stomachache, and fear?

Because of these interconnections, the Emotional Body, the Mental Body, and the limbic system are extremely significant for persons with chronic digestive tract problems. Read about these Process Centers in Chapter 6 and in Part II.

- On the basis of Steps 1 through 3, choose the organs of the gastrointestinal tract that you have discovered to need healing work.

- Place one of your hands over each of the following Process Centers in turn: the Emotional Body (right side of the forehead); Mental Body (left side of the forehead); limbic system (bridge of the nose).

- Place your second hand over each organ in turn (or over the general area in which you are experiencing difficulties).

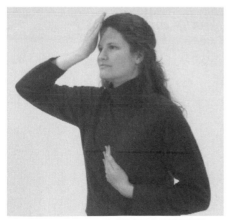

EMOTIONAL BODY AND CARDIAC SPHINCTER

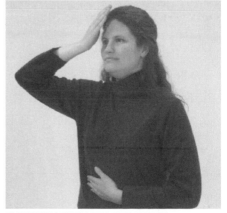

EMOTIONAL BODY AND DUODENUM

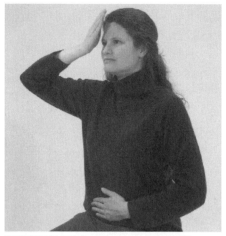

EMOTIONAL BODY AND SMALL INTESTINE

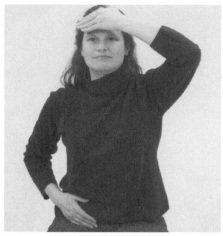

EMOTIONAL BODY AND ILEOCECAL VALVE

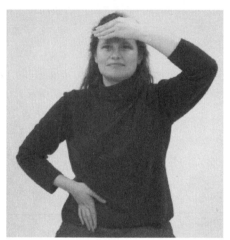

EMOTIONAL BODY AND ASCENDING COLON

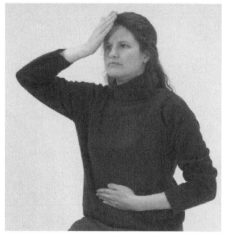

EMOTIONAL BODY AND TRANSVERSE COLON

Hold each of these combinations for as much time as it takes to completely heal these regions.

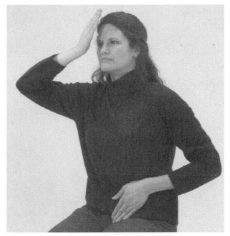

EMOTIONAL BODY AND DESCENDING COLON

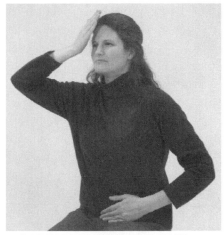

EMOTIONAL BODY AND SIGMOID COLON

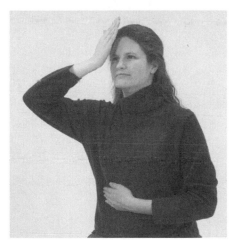

EMOTIONAL BODY AND LIVER

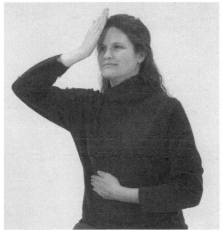

EMOTIONAL BODY AND GALL BLADDER

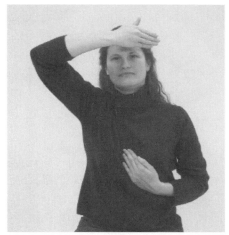

MENTAL BODY AND CARDIAC SPHINCTER

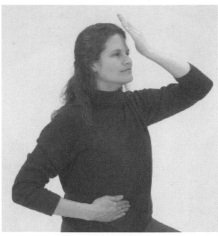

MENTAL BODY AND DUODENUM

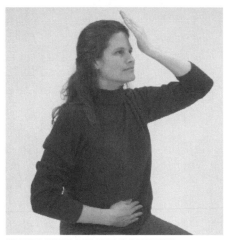

MENTAL BODY AND SMALL INTESTINE

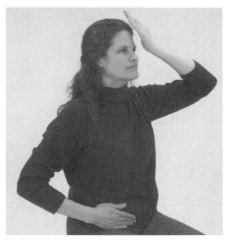

MENTAL BODY AND ILEOCECAL VALVE

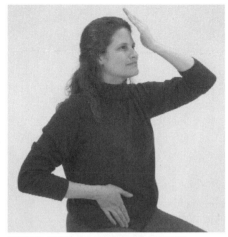

MENTAL BODY AND ASCENDING COLON

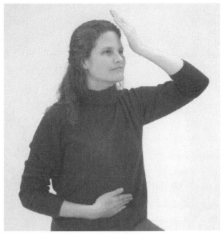

MENTAL BODY AND TRANSVERSE COLON

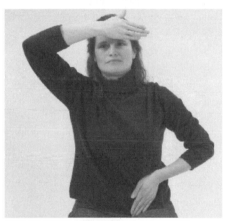

MENTAL BODY AND DESCENDING COLON

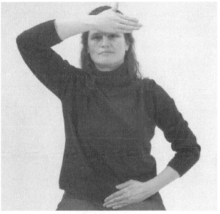

MENTAL BODY AND SIGMOID COLON

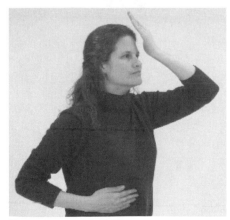

MENTAL BODY AND LIVER

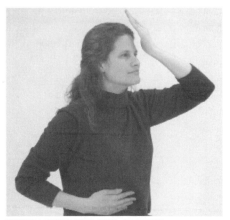

MENTAL BODY AND GALL BLADDER

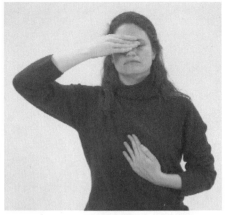

LIMBIC SYSTEM AND CARDIAC SPHINCTER

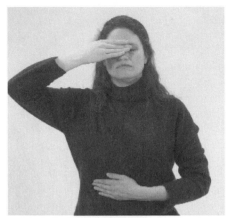

LIMBIC SYSTEM AND DUODENUM

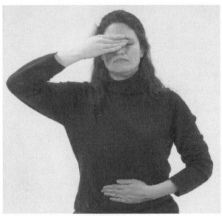

LIMBIC SYSTEM AND SMALL INTESTINE

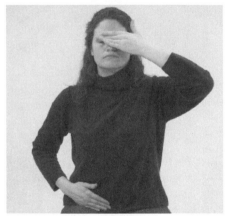

LIMBIC SYSTEM AND ILEOCECAL VALVE

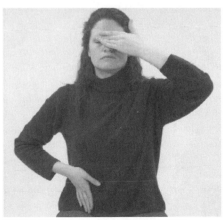

LIMBIC SYSTEM AND ASCENDING COLON

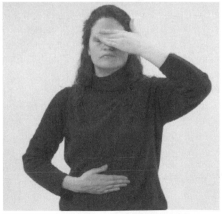

LIMBIC SYSTEM AND TRANSVERSE COLON

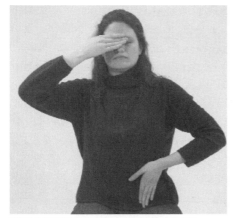

LIMBIC SYSTEM AND DESCENDING COLON

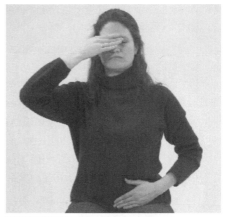

LIMBIC SYSTEM AND SIGMOID COLON

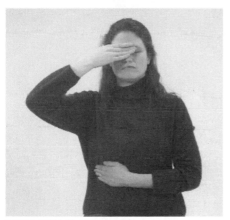

LIMBIC SYSTEM AND LIVER

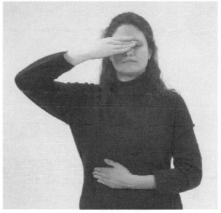

LIMBIC SYSTEM AND GALL BLADDER

ANKLE: Talus (top front part of the ankle joint)
Bone Bruises

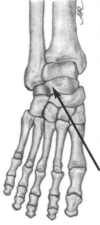

The most common area of pain is the top, front part of the ankle. Place one hand over the talus and lower tibia. Trauma often causes "bone bruises." These can be discovered with high density MRI investigation. A bone bruise has been defined as a microtrabecular fracture, i.e. a fracture that occurs along a network within the bone. These bone bruises on the talus are extremely painful and limit ankle motion.

Talus

STEP 1

- Place one hand on the ankle, covering the talus.

- Place a second hand under the low back, to contact the ureters.

Pain and inflammation will typically subside within an hour for an acute injury, within three hours for a chronic problem.

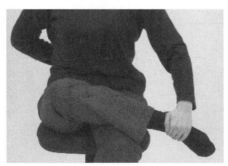

SUPERIOR/ANTERIOR TALUS AND URETERS

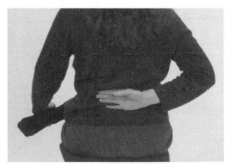

SUPERIOR/ANTERIOR TALUS AND URETERS
(REAR VIEW)

STEP 2

- When the pain subsides, keep one hand over the talus, or where the ankle hurts.

- Place the second hand over the heart.

The ankle will begin to heal. Standing will become less painful. One hour is sufficient for an acute injury. Maintain contact for a total of three hours (does not need to be consecutive) for chronic problems.

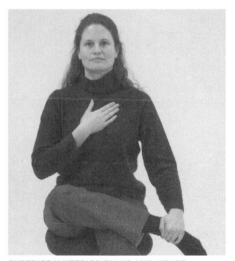

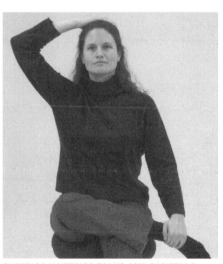

SUPERIOR/ANTERIOR TALUS AND HEART   **SUPERIOR/ANTERIOR TALUS AND PARIETALS**

STEP 3

- When the discomfort has further subsided but walking is still difficult, keep one hand over the talus, or where the ankle hurts.

- Place the second hand on top of the head, over the parietals.

Walking will become less painful. One hour is sufficient for an acute injury. Maintain contact for a total of three hours (does not need to be consecutive) for chronic problems.

STEP 4

If there are any remaining ankle problems, for example if the ankle still hurts or if there are still difficulties in walking, consider using the other Process Centers described in this book.

- Read about the Process Centers as outlined and explained in Chapter 6.
- Choose the Process Centers you want to explore and read about them in Part II.
- Place one hand on the talus or where the ankle hurts.
- Place the second hand on the Process Center of your choice.

You can continue this process for as long as you wish. There are no contraindications; there are no precautions.

ANKLE: Medial Malleolus (inside of the ankle joint)
Pronated Feet (flat feet)

A common area of ankle pain is at the medial malleolus. This pain occurs often with persons with flat feet (pronated feet). Pain at the medial malleolus does not occur as often with persons with high arches. There is a strain of the ligaments in the region of the medial malleolus.

Medial
Malleolus

STEP 1

- Place one hand over the medial malleolus.
- Place the second hand under the low back, to contact the ureters.

Pain and inflammation will typically subside within an hour for an acute injury, within three hours for a chronic problem.

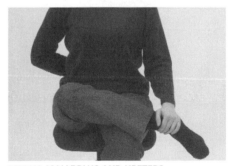

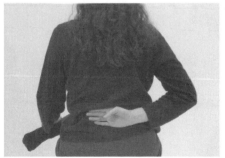

MEDIAL MALLEOLUS AND URETERS   **MEDIAL MALLEOLUS AND URETERS (REAR VIEW)**

STEP 2

- Once the ankle pain subsides, keep one hand over the medial malleolus, or over the ankle where it hurts.
- Place the second hand over the heart.

The ankle will begin to heal. Standing will become less painful. One hour is sufficient for an acute injury. Maintain contact for a total of three hours (does not need to be consecutive) for chronic problems.

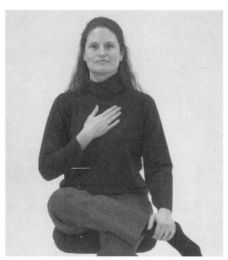

MEDIAL MALLEOLUS AND HEART

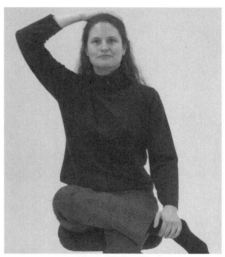

MEDIAL MALLEOLUS AND PARIETALS

STEP 3

- Once the pain has subsided but walking is still difficult, keep one hand over the ankle.
- Place the second hand on top of the head, over the parietals.

Walking will become less painful. One hour is sufficient for an acute injury.

STEP 4

If there are any remaining problems, for example, if the ankle still hurts or if there are still difficulties in walking, consider using the other Process Centers described in this book.

- Read about the Process Centers as outlined and explained in Chapter 6.
- Choose the Process Centers you want to explore and read about them in Part II.
- Place one hand on the medial malleolus or where the ankle hurts.
- Place the second hand on the Process Center of your choice.

You can continue this process for as long as you wish. There are no contraindications; there are no precautions.

ANKLE: Lateral Malleolus (outside of the ankle joint)
Supinated Feet (high arches)

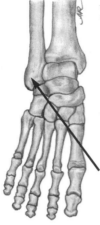

A common area of ankle pain is at the lateral malleolus. This pain occurs often with persons with high arches (supinated feet). Pain at the lateral malleolus does not occur as often with persons with flat feet. People with high arches tend to re-sprain their ankle joints. There is often significant long-term swelling at the lateral malleolus, which commonly responds well to this therapy.

Lateral
Malleolus

STEP 1

• Place one hand over the lateral malleolus.

• Place the second hand under the low back, to contact the ureters.

Pain and inflammation will typically subside within an hour for an acute injury, within three hours for a chronic problem.

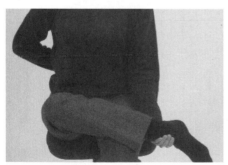

LATERAL MALLEOLUS AND URETERS

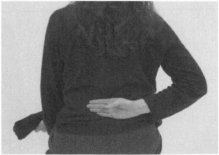

LATERAL MALLEOLUS AND URETERS (REAR VIEW)

- Once the ankle pain subsides, keep one hand over the lateral malleolus, or over the ankle where it hurts.
- Place the second hand over the heart.

The ankle will begin to heal. Standing will become less painful. One hour is sufficient for an acute injury. Maintain contact for a total of three hours (does not need to be consecutive) for chronic problems. Walking will become less painful.

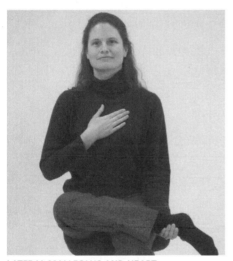 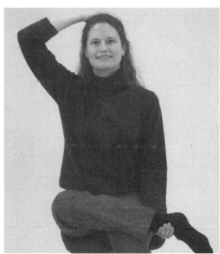

LATERAL MALLEOLUS AND HEART   **LATERAL MALLEOLUS AND PARIETALS**

- Once the pain has subsided, but when walking is still difficult, keep one hand over the ankle.
- Place the second hand on top of the head, over the parietals.

STEP 4

If there are any remaining problems, for example, if the ankle still hurts or there are still difficulties in walking, consider using the other Process Centers in this book.

- Read about the Process Centers as outlined and explained in Chapter 6.
- Choose the Process Centers you want to explore and read about them in Part II.
- Place one hand on the lateral malleolus or where the ankle hurts.
- Place the second hand on the Process Center of your choice.

You can continue this process for as long as you wish. There are no contraindications; there are no precautions.

LOW BACK
Problems with L5 and S1 Vertebrae, the Sacroiliac Joint, the Sacral Plexus

There is so much to say about low back pain. Eight of ten Americans will suffer from it at some point during their lifetime. Eighty-five percent of all spinal surgery is performed between the fifth lumbar vertebra and the first sacral vertebra. This region is called the lumbosacral junction. It has confused health care practitioners, irritated adults who have pain and disability, and confounded researchers. Indeed, the most important aspect of the low back is this region between L5 and S1. The discs between these vertebrae are vulnerable. The nerve roots become compressed and cause low back pain as well as pain in the buttocks and legs. But Neurofascial Process or good manual therapy can definitely alleviate these symptoms.

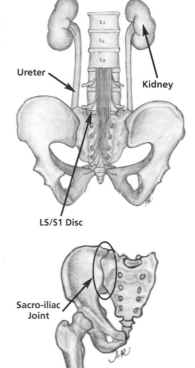

Another source of low back pain is the sacroiliac. This joint also responds to manual therapy. Compression of nerves in this region is a major source of foot pain, knee pain, leg pain, and buttock pain.

Still another cause of back pain is the kidneys. Occasionally, both kidneys together cause pain. However, often a single kidney will be found to be the culprit. When the kidneys are the problem, or part of the problem, the only symptom may be back pain, rather than any other indication of kidney problem. When the kidney is the source, the low back pain will be at the bottom of the rib cage, slightly higher than when the cause is a sacroiliac or L5/S1 problem.

Finally, the ureters may be the sole or partial cause of low back pain. When the ureters are the cause of pain, there is always a problem of toxicity in the body. Toxic drainage is compromised. There may be other signs and indications of ill health.

Since the lumbosacral junction (including the disc and nerves between L5 and S1) is the greatest cause of low back pain, it is sensible to tackle therapy for this region separately.

STEP 1

Usually there is inflammation at the lumbosacral junction. The disc may be protruding or even herniated. The nerves may be compressed and causing pain in the buttocks or legs. If you or someone you know is considering surgery for these reasons, perform the following treatment first.

Over fifty percent of persons who undergo surgery in this region continue to suffer some of the pain, and their disability still remains thereafter. If this is the case, perform this treatment as soon as possible after surgery.

- Place one hand over the lumbosacral junction. Maintain good contact. Often it is easier to use the assistance of another person.

- Place the second hand behind the low back, over the ureters.

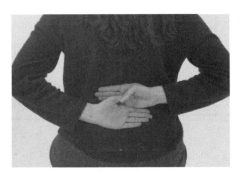
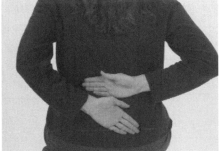

L5, S1, AND URETERS   SACROILIAC JOINT, SACRAL PLEXUS, AND URETERS

Maintain contact (does not need to be consecutive)for as long as you feel benefits. When there is an acute low back pain attack, often the pain will dissolve within one hour. When there is a history of chronic low back pain, even ten hours may not be enough to experience all the effects of Neurofascial Process to the ureters. If you have had surgery, whether recently or many years ago, you may experience benefits from this treatment for many months, if you perform the treatment daily for one hour or more over a period of several months.

There are no precautions or contraindications.

STEP 2

Whenever there is a history of low back pain, consider that there is probably a problem of the sacroiliac joints. Also, consider that there is probably a problem of the sacral plexus.

- Contact the sacroiliac joint and the sacral plexus together with the ureters. You may require the assistance of another person.

STEP 3

When the symptoms of low back pain are decreasing, and movement is improving, consider continuing the healing process for the low back by using the heart as a Process Center.

The contact must be good, so perform this treatment thoroughly.

- First contact first the lumbosacral junction together with the heart.

- Then contact the sacroiliac joint and the sacral plexus with the heart.

The contact with the heart can continue for a hundred hours. When there is a considerable history, you will want to consider this as a long-term project.

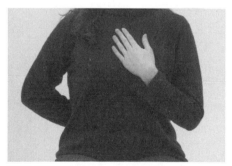
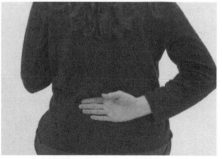

L5/S1 AND HEART   SACROILIAC JOINT, SACRAL PLEXUS, AND HEART

STEP 4

There is *always* a contribution of the limbic system in healing of the low back. Consider contact between all areas of the low back—the lumbosacral junction and the sacroiliac joint and the sacral plexus—with the bridge of the nose. After this treatment you will feel looser than you have in years. You will stop walking like a board, no longer fearful a jolt will compromise the safety you have secured for your low back. Have patience. You will need to continue with the process long enough to gain some real stability for your low back.

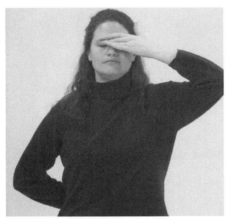

L5/S1 AND LIMBIC SYSTEM

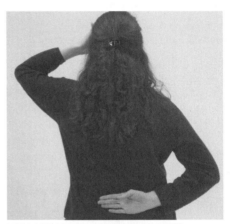

L5/S1 AND LIMBIC SYSTEM (REAR VIEW)

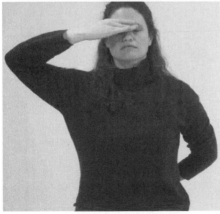

SACROILIAC JOINT, SACRAL PLEXUS, AND LIMBIC SYSTEM

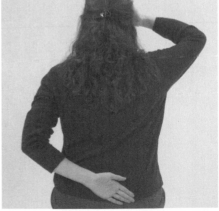

SACROILIAC JOINT, SACRAL PLEXUS, AND LIMBIC SYSTEM (REAR VIEW)

To work with the connection between the limbic system and the lumbosacral junction:

- Place one hand over the lumbosacral junction.
- Place the second hand on the bridge of the nose. Maintain good contact.

To work with the connection between the limbic system and the sacroiliac joint and sacral plexus:

- Place one hand under the sacroiliac joint and sacral plexus.
- Place the second hand on the bridge of the nose. Maintain good contact.

STEP 5

There is *always* fear associated with low back pain. Often the fear regards security, with endless concerns like these: with this pain how can I go to school? How can I go to work? If I don't show up again I may lose my job. What if I need to pick up my child? How can I hide from my spouse any longer that I cannot enjoy our relationship because I am afraid to upset the safety network I have provided for my low back when I don't move it? Will I always have low back pain? Do I really need surgery? I saw what happened when my neighbor had back surgery. What am I going to do? I really cannot stand this pain any longer!

Consider your fears associated with low back pain, particularly with low back pain and issues about security, diminishment of quality of life, and changes in lifestyle.

- Use the kidneys as a Process Center.

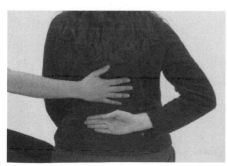

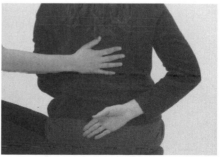

L5/S1 AND KIDNEYS

SACROILIAC JOINT, SACRAL PLEXUS, AND KIDNEYS

Occasionally it is difficult to reach high enough to maintain contact with the kidneys. Ask for assistance from a friend or family member. You can even offer to perform Neurofascial Process for them, if they will help you with your treatment.

Healing may continue for a total of ten or more hours of contact (does not need to be consecutive) with the kidneys.

STEP 6

All of the Process Centers are beneficial for continued healing of the low back. After the kidneys, no one is less important than the others. While the low back continues to heal, and the symptoms subside, consider continuing with this self-healing process for the low back.

- Read about the Process Centers as outlined and explained in Chapter 6.
- Choose the Process Centers you want to explore and read about them in Part II.
- Place one hand over the low back.
- Place the second hand on the Process Center of your choice.

You can continue this process for as long as you wish. There are no contraindications; there are no precautions.

Low Back
Pain Involving the Kidneys

STEP 1

Pain from the kidneys is higher on the low back than pain from L5/S1, from the sacroiliac joint, and from the sacral plexus. Occasionally there is a real problem with the kidney. Often there is only discomfort, but this can be intense.

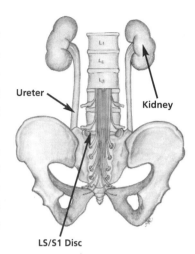

When pain is higher up on the low back, consider making contact with the kidneys and the other Process Centers. The first contact can be the ureters. Often the problem is toxicity within the kidney that requires drainage by the ureters.

- Place one hand on the kidney or kidneys. You may require assistance; it is difficult to stretch so high on the low back and maintain good contact. Good contact is essential.

- Place the second hand behind the low back, on the ureters. You hands may be touching, because the kidneys and ureters are next to each other.

If after one hour there is some decrease in discomfort, continue for as long as the discomfort subsides.

If there is a history of kidney problems, rather than low back pain alone, consider continuing the contact with the ureters for a total of ten to twenty hours (does not need to be consecutive).

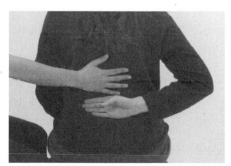

KIDNEY AND URETERS

STEP 2

There is always a healing component connecting the kidneys with the heart that will contribute to healing the kidneys.

- Place one hand on the kidneys.
- Place the second hand on the heart.

When there is a history of chronic or severe kidney dysfunction, you may want to consider this contact for one hour per day for several months.

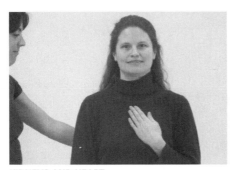

KIDNEYS AND HEART

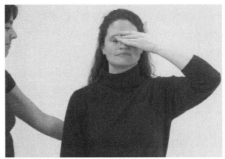

KIDNEYS AND LIMBIC SYSTEM

STEP 3

There is always a history of involvement of the limbic system with kidney problems. There is always a history of involvement of the Emotional Body with kidney problems. There is always a history of involvement of the Mental Body with kidney problems.

- Read in Chapter 6 and in Part II about these Process Centers: the limbic system, the Emotional Body, and the Mental Body as Process Centers.

Typically there is remarkable healing when the kidneys are connected with these Process Centers.

- Place one hand on the kidneys.
- Place the second hand on the bridge of the nose, for contact with the limbic system Process Center.

- Place one hand on the kidneys.
- Place the second hand slightly above the right side of the forehead for contact with the Emotional Body Process Center.

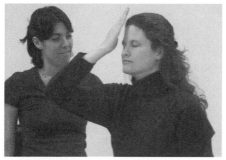 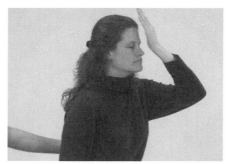

KIDNEYS AND EMOTIONAL BODY   **KIDNEYS AND MENTAL BODY**

- Place one hand on the kidneys.
- Place the second hand slightly above the left side of the forehead for contact with the Mental Body Process Center.

At least one hour of contact for each Process Center above is beneficial. The process can even be applied for longer periods for optimal results.

STEP 4

All of the Process Centers are beneficial for continued healing of the kidneys when they are the cause of low back pain. No one Process Center is less important than the others. While the low back continues to heal and the symptoms are subsiding, consider continuing with the following self-healing processes for the low back.

- Read about the Process Centers as outlined and explained in Chapter 6.
- Choose the Process Centers you want to explore and read about them in Part II.
- Place one hand over the high low back.
- Place the second hand on the Process Center of your choice.

You can continue this process for as long as you wish. There are no contraindications; there are no precautions.

LOW BACK
Pain Involving the Ureters

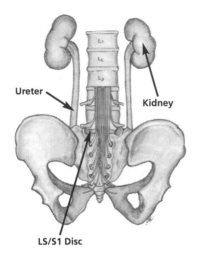

Ureter

Kidney

LS/S1 Disc

The ureters are in the center of the low back and can cause excruciating pain. They connect the kidneys with the bladder, draining toxins into the bladder. The ureters may be considered both as a site for treatment and as a Process Center. As a Process Center, they are the center for toxic drainage. This means that any kind of process in the body involving a drainage of toxins, involves the ureters. Some of these processes would include inflammation and infection.

When the ureters are the primary source of low back pain, there is always a problem of toxicity in the body. The ureters are overworked. They require healing. They need to be connected to all of the other Process Centers. You will benefit from working with each one. Pain will occur less often, will not last as long, and in the end will not be as severe. Occasionally the function of the ureters themselves will improve. When this happens, the toxicity of the body will decrease and general healing will ensue.

Connect the ureters with all of the Process Centers, one at a time or together.

- Place one hand behind the low back, on the ureters.

- Place the second hand over the heart.

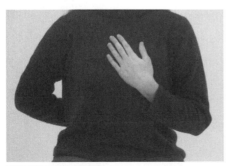

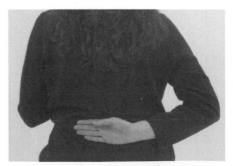

URETERS AND HEART   URETERS AND HEART (REAR VIEW)

- Place one hand behind the low back, on the ureters.
- Place the second hand behind the low back, on the kidneys.

- Place one hand behind the low back, on the ureters.
- Place the second hand over the genital region.

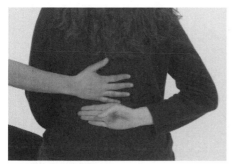

URETERS AND KIDNEYS

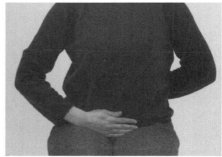

URETERS AND GENITALS

- Place one hand behind the low back, on the ureters.
- Place the second hand on the forehead.

- Place one hand behind the low back, on the ureters.
- Place the second hand on the bridge of the nose.

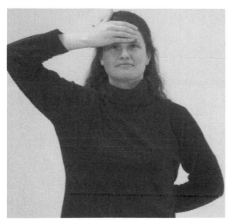

URETERS AND FOREHEAD

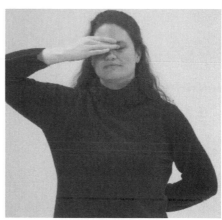

URETERS AND LIMBIC SYSTEM

You can continue this process for as long as you wish. There are no contraindications; there are no precautions.

While the low back continues to heal and the symptoms are subsiding, consider continuing with the other self-healing processes for the low back.

BLADDER
Discomfort; Infection

Bladder infections are common, often giving rise to inflammation at the bladder and causing pain and other sensations in this organ.

Usually this self-healing approach will reduce the discomfort at the bladder. Often the inflammation appears as warmth and swelling. Often the region will become cooler, and the swelling may also subside. Occasionally there is improvement of the bladder infection. If pain and inflammation seem to subside, consider discussing with your physician the option of decreasing your medications.

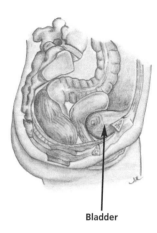

Bladder

STEP 1

- Place one hand over the bladder region. It is directly underneath the pubic bone. Place your hand on top of the pubic bone to contact the bladder.

- Place a second hand under the low back, to contact the ureters.

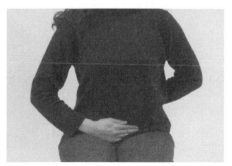

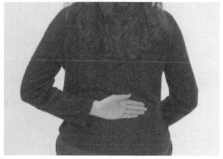

BLADDER AND URETERS   BLADDER AND URETERS (REAR VIEW)

If the bladder inflammation seems to subside after one hour, continue with this technique. This may be an excellent method to reduce bladder discomfort as well as inflammation. Consider up to five hours or more of this treatment (does not need to be consecutive). There are no contraindications and no precautions.

STEP 2

Even when the region of the bladder appears less swollen and less uncomfortable, consider continuing this self-healing process.

• Place one hand over the bladder region.

• Place the second hand on top of the heart.

There are no time limitations. While the symptoms subside, continue for a total of five hours or more.

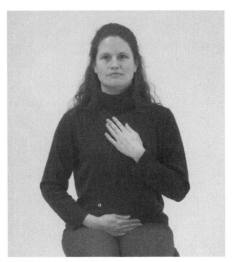

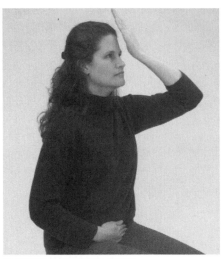

BLADDER AND HEART   **BLADDER AND MENTAL BODY**

STEP 3

When the region of the bladder continues to heal, you may wish to continue with the following self-healing approach.

Thoughts about the bladder often cause us internal stress; therefore, working with the Mental Body as a Process Center together with the bladder is a good idea.

• Read about the Mental Body (frontal region) as a Process Center in Chapter 11.

• Place one hand over the bladder region.

• Place the second hand over the Mental Body.

STEP 4

Sometimes, unbeknownst to us, we have fears about urination that contribute to stress; therefore, working with the kidneys together with the bladder is a good idea.

- Read about the kidneys as a Process Center in Chapter 10.
- Place one hand over the bladder region.
- Place the second hand under the kidneys.

You may want to consider any of your fears associated with the bladder and urination, although to do so is not a requirement.

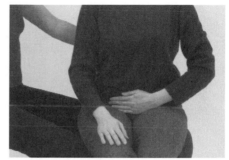

BLADDER AND KIDNEYS

STEP 5

While the bladder continues to heal, there will be less discomfort in the pelvic region. Consider using other Process Centers as you continue with this self-healing process for the bladder.

- Read about the Process Centers as outlined and explained in Chapter 6.
- Choose the Process Centers you want to explore and read about them in Part II.
- Place one hand over the bladder.
- Place the second hand on the Process Center of your choice.

You can continue this process for as long as you wish. There are no contraindications; there are no precautions.

EAR
Earache; Infection; Tinnitus (ringing in the ears)

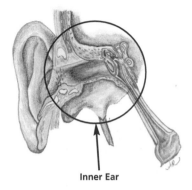

Inner Ear

Infection and/or inflammation in the ear are common problems. The symptoms may vary: pain, buzzing, discomfort, ringing, loud noises, burning, itching, as well as other annoying sensations, even when the doctor has given us a clean bill of health. The following process with the ears is suitable for persons who are diagnosed with infection as well as those who are given the clean bill of health.

STEP 1

- Place one hand over the ear. Do not press hard, yet maintain good contact.
- Place the second hand under the low back, for contact with the ureters.

Continue with these hand placements for at least an hour.

When there is a history of chronic ear infections, or if there are tubes in the ears, with or without a history of antibiotics, continue for at least one session for two straight hours.

When the pain or discomfort starts to subside, continue for up to a total of ten hours (does not need to be consecutive).

There are no contraindications or precautions.

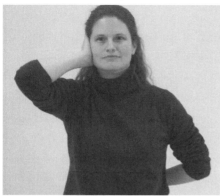
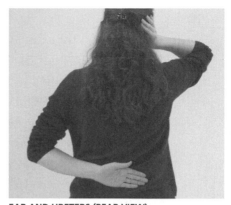

EAR AND URETERS   EAR AND URETERS (REAR VIEW)

STEP 2

When there is a history of recurrent ear infection, the presence of tubes or the incidence of other recent surgeries, consider continuing with the following healing process.

• Place one hand over the ear.

• Place the second hand over the heart.

When there is real dysfunction in and around the ear, it is worthwhile to maintain these contacts for up to ten hours (does not need to be consecutive). If the pain and inflammation subside, continue for as long as you wish.

There are no contraindications or precautions.

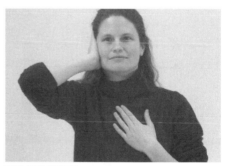

EAR AND HEART

STEP 3

Occasionally we are incapable of remembering what bothers us. If at any time in your life you had ear surgery or experienced some other trauma to the ear, you may have repressed the memories associated with it. If there is a history of trauma, surgery, or other events associated with ears and hearing, consider the following contacts.

- Place one hand over the ear.
- Place the second hand over the bridge of the nose.

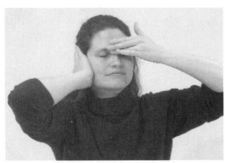

Memories are associated with the limbic system. Contact for the limbic system is at the bridge of the nose. Read about the limbic system as a Process Center in Part II.

EAR AND LIMBIC SYSTEM

STEP 4

While the ear continues to heal, and the symptoms are subsiding, consider continuing with the following self-healing process for the ear.

- Read about the Process Centers as outlined and explained in Chapter 6.
- Choose the Process Centers you want to explore and read about them in Part II.
- Place one hand over the ear.
- Place the second hand on the Process Center of your choice.

You can continue this process for as long as you wish. There are no contraindications; there are no precautions.

ELBOW
Pain

Elbow trauma is common, resulting in sharp throbbing pain, dull aching pain, or pins and needles through the forearm and hand at the moment of the trauma.

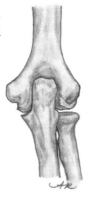

STEP 1

For acute elbow trauma, when the elbow is inflamed, sore, swollen, painful to touch, Neurofascial Process to the ureters is a wonderful first aid.

- Place one hand on the elbow. Try to contact all aspects of the elbow.
- Place the second hand under the low back for contact with the ureters.

It may be difficult to contact the elbow at the same time as you contact on the low back. You may require assistance from another person.

When swelling is acute, hold this contact for one hour. If swelling and pain continue, this process may help if performed for up to a total of five hours (does not need to be consecutive).

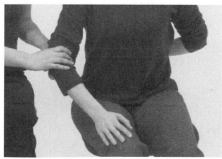

ELBOW AND URETERS

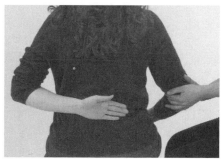

ELBOW AND URETERS (REAR VIEW)

STEP 2

When swelling is gone or almost gone, yet irritation, pain, and limited movement persists, consider continuing with the following process.

- Place one hand on the elbow.
- Place the second hand on the heart.

Continue up to a total of three hours contact. You will probably require the assistance of a second person.

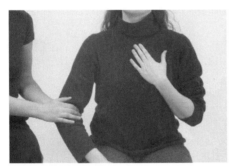

ELBOW AND HEART

STEP 3

While the elbow continues to heal, there will be less discomfort in the arm, and the range of elbow movement will increase. Consider continuing with the following self-healing process for the elbow.

- Read about the Process Centers as outlined and explained in Chapter 6.
- Choose the Process Centers you want to explore and read about them in Part II.
- Place one hand over the elbow.
- Place the second hand on the Process Center of your choice.

You can continue this process for as long as you wish. There are no contraindications; there are no precautions.

EYE
Infection; Blurred Vision; Pain; Other Symptoms

Often there is infection and/or inflammation in the eye, even when your doctor has given you a clean bill of health. The symptoms of infection and/or inflammation may be: pain, blurred vision, seeing double or triple images, irritation, poor visual clarity, depth perception problems, burning, itching, as well as other annoying troubles. The following process with the eyes is suitable both for persons who are diagnosed with infection and those who are given a clean bill of health.

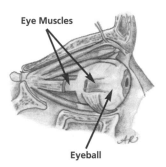

Eye Muscles

Eyeball

STEP 1

- Place one hand over the eye. Do not press hard, yet maintain good contact.
- Place the second hand under the low back for contact with the ureters.

Continue with these hand placements at least for an hour.

When there is a history of chronic eye infection, with or without a history of antibiotics, continue for at least one session for two straight

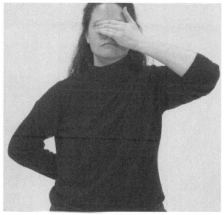

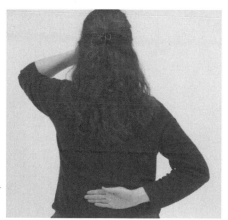

EYE AND URETERS   **EYE AND URETERS (REAR VIEW)**

hours. If the pain, discomfort or other symptoms start to subside, continue for up to a total of ten hours (does not need to be consecutive).

There are no contraindications or precautions.

STEP 2

When there is a history of recurrent eye infection, surgery, or other traumatic events, consider continuing with the following healing process.

- Place one hand over the eye.

- Place the second hand over the heart.

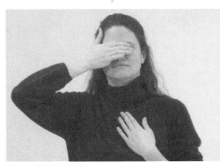

When there are significant problems in and around the eye, it is worthwhile to maintain this contact for up to a total of ten hours (does not need to be consecutive). If the pain and inflammation subside, and vision begins to improve, continue for as long as you wish.

There are no contraindications or precautions.

EYE AND HEART

STEP 3

Often vision is associated with fear. Occasionally this is based on subconscious causes—you are not aware of the cause of the fear. Often the fear is a fear of remembering something you saw, or thought you saw. Consider what would happen if you were able to eliminate the fear associated with vision: you would no longer be afraid of what you might see.

- Read about the kidneys as a Process-Center in Chapter 10.

- Place one hand over the eyes.

- Place the second hand over the kidneys.

Maintain this contact for at least one hour (does not need to be consecutive). When the eye symptoms appear to change, continue for up to a total of five hours.

There are no precautions or contraindications.

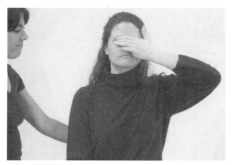

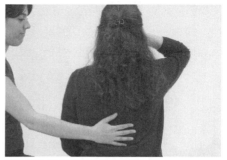

EYE AND KIDNEYS   **EYE AND KIDNEYS (REAR VIEW)**

STEP 4

Occasionally we are incapable of remembering what bothers us. If at any time in your life you had eye surgery, you may have repressed the memories associated with traumatic events such as surgery. If there is a history of trauma, surgery, or other events associated with eyes and seeing, consider applying the following process.

- Read about the limbic system as a Process Center in Chapter 9.
- Place one hand over the eyes.
- Place the second hand over the bridge of the nose.

Memories are associated with the limbic system. Contact with the limbic system can be established at the bridge of the nose.

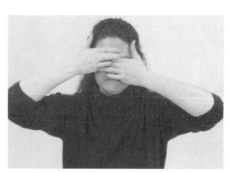

EYE AND LIMBIC SYSTEM

STEP 5

While the eye continues to heal and the symptoms subside, consider continuing with the following self-healing process for the eye.

- Read about the Process Centers as outlined and explained in Chapter 6.
- Choose the Process Centers you want to explore and read about them in Part II.
- Place one hand over the eye.
- Place the second hand on the Process Center of your choice.

You can continue this process for as long as you wish. There are no contraindications; there are no precautions.

HEART
Pain; Coronary Heart Disease; Blood Pressure Problems

Coronary heart disease and heart problems were the leading cause of death in the United States in the year 2000. Of course, people are taking so much medication that it is possible that the medicines used for the treatment of heart problems are the real culprits. The second and fourth causes of death are "iatrogenic," that is physician or medication related. Consider your age. Are you too young to be taking medication? Are you afraid to decrease the medi-

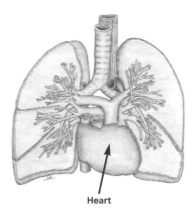

Heart

cation? How many pills do you swallow each day—one pill? Two pills? Five pills? Twelve pills? Are you ready to do something for your heart problem? You can start with this self-healing approach. After you begin to work with it a bit, you may experience less chest pain. Perhaps some of your neck and left arm pain will diminish. Maybe you will stop feeling quite as dizzy or lightheaded. Maybe you will have more movement at your neck, arm, and low back. Perhaps the sores on your leg will start to heal. You only need to do this work and wait and see. You have nothing to lose but time. There are no precautions or contraindications.

STEP 1

Recent medical research shows that there may be a direct connection between heart problems and infection.

- Assume that there may be *some* infection or inflammation that has affected your heart or pericardium (the area around the heart) in the past.
- Place one hand on the heart.
- Place the second hand behind the low back on the ureters.

If you have no history of heart problems, and you want to practice this technique (with the understanding that *you never know how good you will feel until you get there!*) maintain the hand placements for at least one hour. If you have a history of heart problems, blood pressure problems, or any other cardiovascular disorder, maintain these hand placements for at least a total of five hours. If symptoms subside, if you are feeling better in any way, it could be helpful to continue with this hand placement for up to twenty hours or more (in all cases, hours do not need to be consecutive).

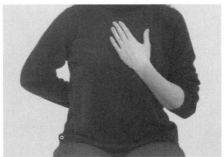

HEART AND URETERS

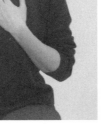

HEART AND URETERS (REAR VIEW)

STEP 2

The frontal lobe of the brain is the Mental Body Process Center. (See Chapter 11.) It has the unique ability to help us process information. Usually, the connection between the heart and the frontal lobe can be extremely conducive to healing.

- Place one hand on the heart.
- Place the second hand on your forehead.

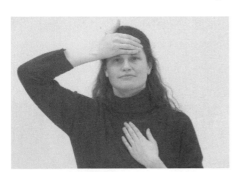

Continue with these hand placements for as long as you continue to feel you are improving. Start with at least one hour. Then continue.

HEART AND FOREHEAD

STEP 3

All of the Process Centers in this book are important for healing the heart. Apply all of the following Process Centers with the heart: Mental Body; Emotional Body; limbic system at the bridge of the nose; kidneys; upper arms; forearms. Start with at least one hour for each of these and continue with the hand placements for as long as you continue to feel you are improving

- Place one hand on the heart.
- For the Mental Body, place the second hand slightly off the left side of the forehead.

- Place one hand on the heart.
- For the Emotional Body, place the second hand slightly off the right forehead.

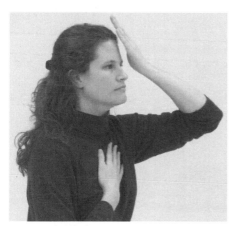
HEART AND MENTAL BODY

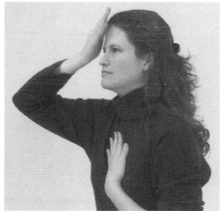
HEART AND EMOTIONAL BODY

- Place one hand on the heart.
- For the limbic system, place the second hand on the bridge of the nose.

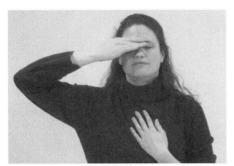

HEART AND LIMBIC SYSTEM

- Place one hand on the heart.
- For the kidneys, place the second hand behind the back, at the level of the bottom ribs, over the kidneys.

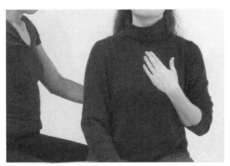 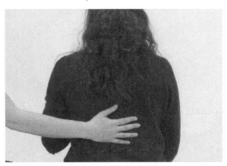

HEART AND KIDNEYS   **HEART AND KIDNEYS (REAR VIEW)**

- Place one hand on the heart.
- For the upper arms, place the second hand on the upper arms, one arm at a time, unless there is assistance from someone else.

- Place one hand on the heart.
- For the forearms, place the second hand on a forearm. When one forearm is completed, contact other forearm.

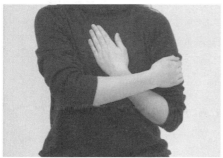 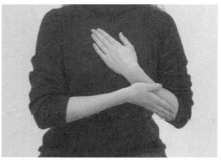

HEART AND UPPER ARM   **HEART AND FOREARM**

For how long should you continue with this treatment of the heart? For the rest of your life! If you have a disease or a severe disorder, you might choose a to combine the heart with a different Process Center every day and treat yourself for an hour a day, every day forever. If a friend or family member has heart problems, you can use multiple hands: one person places a hand on the heart; others have their hands on the other Process Centers respectively. You can perform this treatment for many hours during the day. There are no precautions or contraindications.

HIP
Pain; Post-Surgery

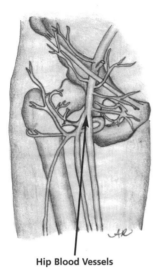

Hip Blood Vessels

Often people experience hip pain when the problem is really with the low back. Similarly, often the hip pain occurs because of problems at the sacroiliac joint. Many persons go for hip surgery because their doctor found problems on X-ray at the hip. Frequently, however, their pain goes away without surgery when they get really good manual therapy for the sacroiliac joint.

If the problem causing the hip pain is really from the hip, then the following procedures will help. When there is pain and swelling as a result of hip surgery—even total hip replacement surgery—the same procedures will help.

Remember: First consider whether there is a problem with your sacroiliac joint and low back. Then proceed to the hip.

STEP 1

- Place one hand over the lateral (side) hip joint.
- Place the second hand behind the low back, in contact with the ureters.

Hip pain is usually chronic. With chronic issues many sessions may be required. If your hip pain *is* chronic, maintain the contact for sessions of at least two hours (does not need to be consecutive). If the movement of the hip improves, or there is even a slight decrease in discomfort, it is worthwhile to continue with these contacts for up to a total of ten hours or more.

If the pain is acute, for example after hip replacement surgery, place hands on the above contact regions for one hour. If the pain and swelling seem to subside, as will usually happen, continue with this contact for one hour a day for at least three months following surgery.

STEP 2

Occasionally there is a problem at the front of the hip region that is *not* because of the hip joint. Sometimes the problem is an inguinal or femoral hernia (an out-pouching of the femoral vessels or femoral nerve through the inguinal canal). Sometimes there is a problem of "femoral artery insufficiency," which means the blood flow through the femoral artery is compromised. When that is the case, there may be some hair loss in the lower part of the leg. Sometimes there are sores on the leg. When this is the situation, it is better to contact the front of the hip region and the groin area rather than the hip joint itself.

- Place one hand over the anterior (front) hip joint.
- Place the second hand behind the low back, in contact with the ureters.

Consider maintaining these contacts for as long as you find the hip is continuing to improve.

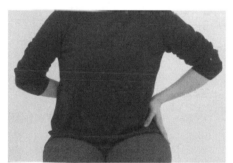

LATERAL HIP AND URETERS

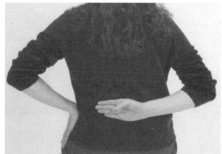

LATERAL HIP AND URETERS (REAR VIEW)

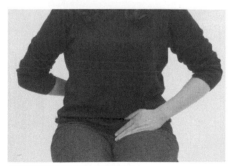

ANTERIOR HIP AND URETERS

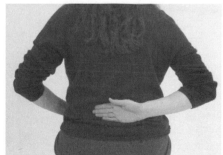

ANTERIOR HIP AND URETERS (REAR VIEW)

STEP 4

Once the hip is feeling better from contact with the ureters, proceed to work with contact with the heart. If the hip joint problem is chronic, often ten or more hours of Neurofascial Process to the heart will help.

- Place one hand on the hip joint.
- Place the second hand on the heart.

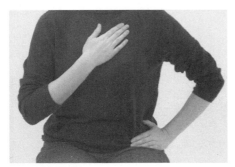

HIP AND HEART

STEP 5

While the hip continues to heal and the symptoms subside, consider continuing with the following self-healing process for the hip.

- Read about the Process Centers as outlined and explained in Chapter 6.
- Choose the Process Centers you want to explore and read about them in Part II.
- Place one hand over the hip.
- Place the second hand on the Process Center of your choice.

You can continue this process for as long as you wish. There are no contraindications; there are no precautions.

KNEE
Pain; Sports Injuries

The knee is responsible for many functions, of which the initiation of walking is the most important. Knee problems are not as prevalent as low back pain, yet in sports contexts many common problems involving the knee do arise.

The knee is often difficult to treat because it is a complex joint. One problem is with the femoralpatellar joint, which is between the patella (knee cap) and the femur bone. The cartilage behind the patella breaks down, and tremendous pain can occur. This cartilage, however, can regenerate with proper manual therapy such as Neurofascial Process.

Another common problem occurs at the lateral collateral ligament at the outside of the knee joint. Sprains can cause tears and irritations of this joint ligament. Sports injuries frequently happen to it, with pain and inflammation as results.

The most common problem of the knee occurs at the medial collateral ligament, which is associated with the meniscus. A sprain of this ligament will cause pressure and strain of the meniscus. It is one of the more common causes of surgery.

The cruciate ligaments, especially the anterior cruciate ligament, are also common sites of sports injuries.

The popliteal fossa is also a common area of pain and swelling. Often there are problems of arterial flow, vein return, and lymph drainage. When the back of the knee—the popliteal fossa—is swollen and hot, consider this region for treatment.

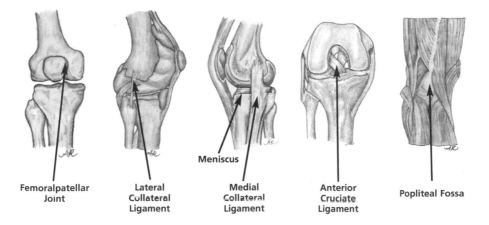

Femoralpatellar
Joint

Lateral
Collateral
Ligament

Meniscus

Medial
Collateral
Ligament

Anterior
Cruciate
Ligament

Popliteal Fossa

STEP 1

Always use Neurofascial Process to the ureters for treatment of acute pain and inflammation. Whatever the cause, whether there was a sport injury, or after surgery (meniscus, total knee replacement or some other operation), this is the very best first aid. If there is also a question of infection of the knee, this is the treatment of choice.

• Place one hand on the knee at the site of pain or the surgery site.

• Place the second hand behind the low back, on the ureters.

If the injury is acute and severe, start with one hour of contact with the knee joint and the ureters. Continue up to three hours. If the injury is chronic, start with three hours. Then continue up to a total of fifteen hours. If the pain and swelling occurs after surgery, start with a minimum total of five hours (in all cases, hours to not need to be consecutive). If one or more hours of treatment per day is performed for three months after surgery, the postsurgical results are often remarkable. Neurofascial Process attains remarkable results with knee problems.

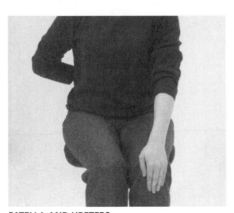
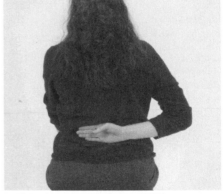

PATELLA AND URETERS   **PATELLA AND URETERS (REAR VIEW)**

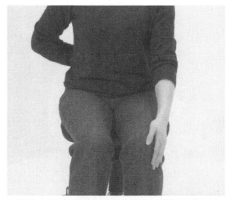

LATERAL COLLATERAL LIGAMENT AND URETERS

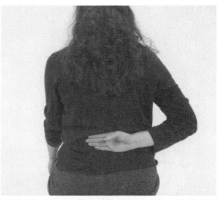

LATERAL COLLATERAL LIGAMENT AND URETERS
(REAR VIEW)

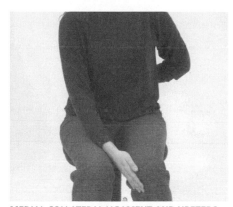

MEDIAL COLLATERAL LIGAMENT AND URETERS

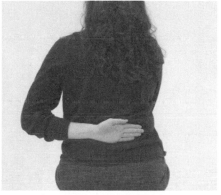

MEDIAL COLLATERAL LIGAMENT AND URETERS
(REAR VIEW)

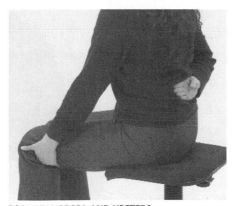

POPLITEAL FOSSA AND URETERS

STEP 2

If the knee is healing but there seems to be a plateau with changes in pain and disability, consider continuing with heart contact.

- Place one hand on the knee.
- Place the second hand over the heart.

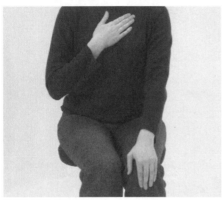

Continue for up to a total of fifteen hours (does not need to be consecutive) if symptoms are improving.

KNEE AND HEART

STEP 3

Even when there appear to be no issues related to the surgery, traumatic events may have occurred and been repressed. Having one's knee cut into is similar to losing a vital organ. Fears associated with getting through surgery at the knee are often more significant than one may recognize. It is important to address these fears to continue the healing process.

- Place one hand on the knee.
- Place the second hand over the kidneys.

Continue these contacts for as long as the knee continues to heal. This may be up to a total of twenty hours (does not need to be consecutive) over a period of a month or more.

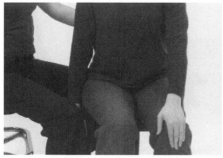

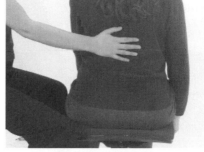

KNEE AND KIDNEYS   **KNEE AND KIDNEYS (REAR VIEW)**

STEP 4

When trauma is associated with the knee, whether from surgery or a car accident or a sports injury, survival instincts surface. The limbic system will influence behaviors. People do not understand why their behaviors are no longer characteristic. They experience low tolerance to illness, low patience, and a low threshold for stress.

An exceptional process to use after knee trauma is making contact between the knee and the bridge of the nose. The bridge of the nose is the contact point for the limbic system.

When the limbic system helps in the knee's healing, often it can be a most remarkable process. You may find the knee continues to heal for months only by maintaining contact with the bridge of the nose. Occasionally this success with contact with the limbic system may be an indication that the bridge of the nose should be used for other areas of discomfort in the body.

- Read about the limbic system as a Process Center in Chapter 9.

- Place one hand on the knee.

- Place the second hand over the bridge of the nose, maintaining good contact.

There are no precautions or contraindications.

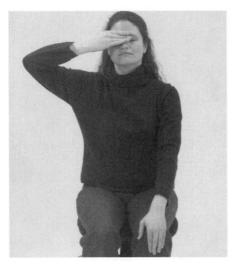

KNEE AND LIMBIC SYSTEM

STEP 5

Often the other Process Centers will have a beneficial effect on the
healing of the knee. Certainly contact with the Emotional Body, the
Mental Body, the forehead, and the parietals are all very beneficial.
While the knee continues to heal and the symptoms subside, consider
continuing with the following self-healing process for the knee.

The first Process Centers to consider are the ones listed above: the
Emotional Body, the Mental Body, the forehead, and the parietals.

- Read about the Process Centers as outlined and explained in Chapter
  6.
- Choose the Process Centers you want to explore.
- Place one hand over the knee.
- Place the second hand on the Process Center of your choice.

You can continue this process for as long as you wish. There are no
contraindications; there are no precautions.

LEARNING DISABILITIES
Dyslexia; Problems with Cognition, Attention, Concentration

There are many voices in America today crying out, "Stop poisoning our children." Prozac for children under the age of four years old? Paxil for teenagers and younger so that they can socialize? Ritalin for children and adolescents of all ages, toxic beyond words? What has happened to our society? When did we lose our per-

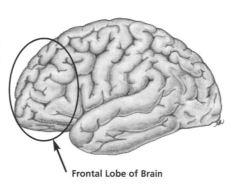

Frontal Lobe of Brain

spective? Why are we not offered other options, such as cognitive and emotional therapies? God help us, for we are abusing our children with drugs for our own selfish purposes.

Many unanswered questions arise when our children do not learn as we expect them to do. What is a learning disability? Who should decide when a child has one? What is mental capacity? Why are the children not paying attention? Where is their concentration? Why can they not read, write, do arithmetic?

Neurofascial Process for frontal lobe healing should be tried whenever question regarding learning problems arise, before subjecting a child to toxic medications. The *frontal lobe* is the region of the brain associated with intelligence, judgment, perception, attention, and concentration.

When a child has a problem like the above, perhaps there is a problem at the frontal lobe.

STEP 1

- Place one hand on the forehead.
- Place the second hand behind the low back, on the ureters.

Maintain contact for a total of five hours (does not need to be consecutive).

STEP 2

- Place one hand on the forehead.
- Place the second hand on the heart.

Maintain contact for a total of five hours (does not need to be consecutive).

STEP 3

- Place one hand on the forehead.
- Place the second hand on the liver.

Maintain contact for a total of five hours (does not need to be consecutive).

STEP 3

- Place one hand on the forehead.
- Place the second hand on the kidneys.

Maintain contact for a total of five hours (does not need to be consecutive).

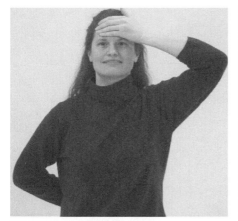

FOREHEAD AND URETERS

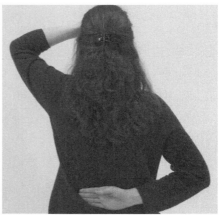

FOREHEAD AND URETERS (REAR VIEW)

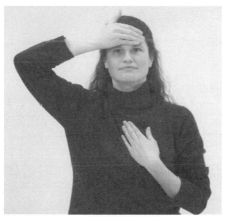

FOREHEAD AND HEART

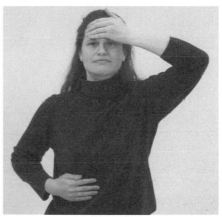

FOREHEAD AND LIVER

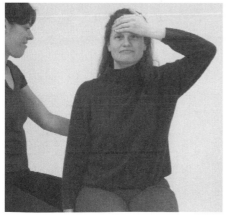

FOREHEAD AND KIDNEYS

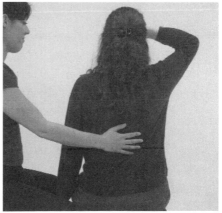

FOREHEAD AND KIDNEYS (REAR VIEW)

STEP 4

- Place one hand on the forehead.
- Place the second hand on the spleen.

Maintain contact for a total of five hours (does not need to be consecutive).

STEP 5

- Place one hand on the forehead.
- Place the second hand on the abdomen, below the belly button.

Maintain contact for a total of five hours (does not need to be consecutive).

STEP 6

- Place one hand on the forehead.
- Place the second hand on the genital region, with a focus on the uterus or prostate.

Maintain contact for a total of five hours (does not need to be consecutive).

There are many recommendations for children with learning disabilities.

First recommendation: Check their vision! If they do not see perfectly *without glasses,* use the treatment protocol for the eyes (presented earlier).

Second recommendation: Check their hearing. If they appear to have any form of hearing deficit, or a history of ear infections, use the treatment protocol for the ears (presented earlier).

Third recommendation: Watch their diet. Food allergies, sinus problems, or other dysfunctions could be the cause of their learning disabilities. Often the learning disability can be corrected for life without drugs. Do not give up hope. Look in your local bookstore for all of the wonderful opportunities to assess the reasons for learning disabilities. Find a nutritionist who can help choose correct foods.

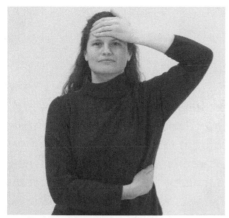

FOREHEAD AND SPLEEN

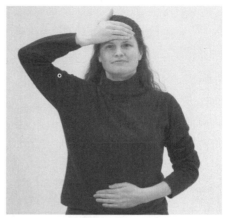

FOREHEAD AND ABDOMEN

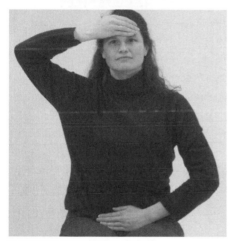

FOREHEAD AND GENITAL REGION

NECK
Pain; Neck Disc Problems

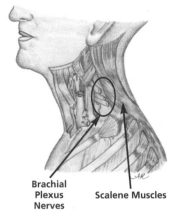

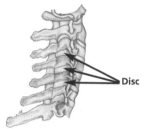

Brachial Plexus Nerves   **Scalene Muscles**

Disc

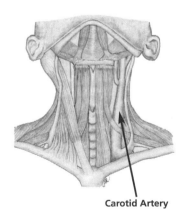

Carotid Artery

Neck pain is a common ailment. Clinical evidence suggests that a lot of neck pain stems from the low back. When the low back is stuck, the neck is stuck. There are seven vertebrae in the neck. The most common problems occur at the fifth vertebra. Often there is a bulging disc at the fifth vertebra. When the disc refers pain down the arm, this is called *cervical syndrome*.

The muscles at the side of the neck are called the scalenes. A common problem called the *scalene syndrome* occurs when the scalene muscles compress the nerves called the brachial plexus.

Sometimes disc problems cause pain at the back of the neck; often the pain from disc herniation (when the disk beneath the vertebra is out-pouching and causing pressure on the spinal cord) is at the side of the neck.

Three vital blood vessels at the side of the neck are the comm on carotid artery, the external carotid artery, and the internal carotid artery. Occasionally severe neck pain is caused by compression of these arteries.

STEP 1

To relieve neck pain, it is good to hold both sides of the neck as well as the back of the neck. If you are limited in time, place your hand on the side of the neck that hurts more, or on the back of the neck.

• Place one hand on your neck.

• Place the second hand on your heart.

If you have a chronic or severe neck problem, maintain hand placements for up to a total of three hours (does not need to be consecutive).

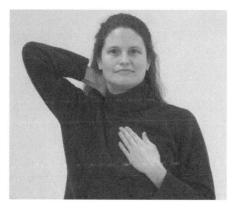 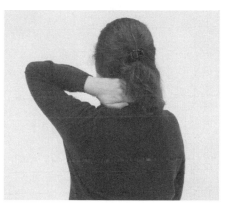

NECK AND HEART   **NECK AND HEART (REAR VIEW)**

STEP 2

If you have headaches as well as neck pain, perhaps there is a carotid artery problem.

- Place one hand on the side of your neck.
- Place the second hand over your heart.

As the neck pain subsides, continue with these hand placements for up to a total of three hours (does not need to be consecutive).

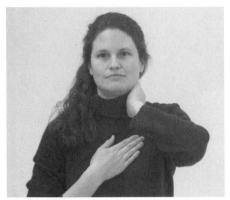
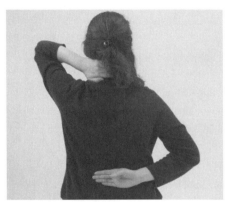

SIDE OF NECK AND HEART   **NECK AND URETERS**

STEP 3

Consider past events. Did you have surgery when you were a child? For example, did you have your tonsils removed? Did you experience discomfort while swallowing? Were you ever seriously ill as a child? Also ask yourself whether your lymph nodes are swollen?

In the case of past surgery or infection, use the ureters as a Process Center.

- Place one hand on your neck.
- Place the second hand behind your low back, on the ureters.

If your history of neck discomfort is mild, one hour of treatment may be enough. If you have a history of serious throat pain or other neck or throat problems, continue for up to five hours (does not need to be consecutive).

STEP 4

As the neck continues to heal and the symptoms are subsiding, consider continuing with the following self-healing process for the neck.

All of the Process Centers are important. You will benefit from each one. Pain will occur less often, will not last as long, and after some time, will not be as severe. There will be more movement of the neck.

- Read about the Process Centers as outlined and explained in Chapter 6.
- Choose the Process Centers you want to explore and read about them in Part II.
- Place one hand over the neck.
- Place the second hand on the Process Center of your choice.

You can continue this process for as long as you wish. There are no contraindications; there are no precautions.

PROSTATE
Pain; Prostatitis

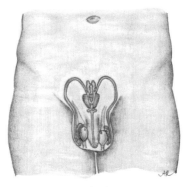

**Male Reproductive Organs
and Genital Region**

The incidence of prostate problems in the USA is enormous. Men have bladder problems that cause constrictions around the urethra. When the urethra is compressed, so are the other vessels of the penis. When the genital vessels in the penis are compressed, there is a reflux of urine back up into the prostate. The prostate becomes inflamed from the back flow of urine. This is only one of many possible reasons for prostatitis.

STEP 1

Inflammation and infection are significant, causing prostate pain and dysfunction. Begin to heal the prostate and reduce the swelling and inflammation with the ureters as a Process Center.

- Place one hand over the prostate, which is slightly above the pubis bone.
- Place the second hand behind the low back, on the ureters.

If the problem is severe or long-term, maintain this hand placement for up to a total of twenty hours (does not need to be consecutive). If there is a diagnosis of prostatitis, certainly there is no reason to stop this treatment if symptoms are subsiding. There are no precautions or contraindications.

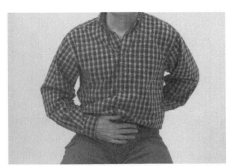

PROSTATE AND URETERS

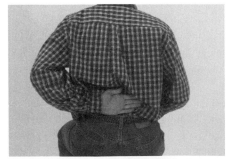

PROSTATE AND URETERS (REAR VIEW)

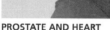

Once the inflammation has subsided and the symptoms are less severe, the healing of the prostate can begin. Use the heart as a Process Center for healing.

- Place one hand on the genital area, over the prostate.
- Place the second hand over the heart.

Even if the symptoms are much diminished, continue for additional hours with this hand placement. Healing of the prostate cannot be overdone. Continue for a total of five, ten, fifteen, or twenty or more hours.

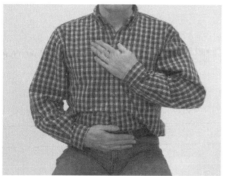 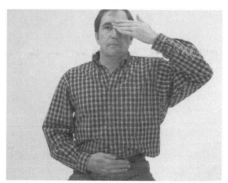

PROSTATE AND HEART   **PROSTATE AND LIMBIC SYSTEM**

STEP 3

Often there is some atypical aggressive behavior associated with male hormones because of prostate problems. If you have indications that you are overly aggressive—perhaps more stressed than you would like; if you are intolerant and impatient—perhaps with a low anger and rage threshold: consider using the bridge of the nose as a Process Center. Read about the limbic system as a Process Center in this book. The bridge of the nose is the hand placement for the limbic system.

Ask yourself: Are you often impatient? Do you tend to get angry at your family, friends, or coworkers? Are you often stressed? This treatment could help you and your prostate!

- Place one hand over the genital region, focusing on the prostate.
- Place the second hand on the bridge of the nose, with good contact.

This hand placement can be maintained for as long as desired. While symptoms are subsiding in the pelvic region, perhaps you may find your behavior is also changing. Perform this treatment for at least one hour.

STEP 4

Allow yourself to continue to heal the prostate and genital region. Your pain and signs of inflammation may subside. Perhaps your total health and well-being have been influenced. It is worth your while to continue with this treatment. While the genital region continues to heal and the symptoms subside, consider continuing with this self-healing process for the genital region.

All of the Process Centers are important. You will benefit from each one. Perhaps many male functions will become less uncomfortable.

- Read about the Process Centers as outlined and explained in Chapter 6.
- Choose the Process Centers you want to explore.
- Place one hand over the prostate and genital region.
- Place the second hand on the Process Center of your choice.

You can continue this process for as long as you wish. There are no contraindications; there are no precautions.

SCIATICA

Usually when there is sciatica, there is also a low back problem. Look at the section of this book on protocols for the low back. Use this approach for all the areas of the low back mentioned: the lumbosacral junction and the sacroiliac joint and the sacral plexus are all important landmarks. When you complete treatment for these as described in this book, proceed with this section on the sciatic nerve.

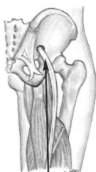

Sciatic Nerve

The sciatic nerve comes out of the fourth and fifth lumbar spaces. It often receives fibers from the sacral plexus. Then it moves behind the ilium, underneath the gluteal muscle and the piriformis muscle, and is often compressed by these muscles. A very vulnerable spot on the sciatic nerve is underneath these muscles, in the middle of the buttocks.

STEP 1

To decrease spasm of the muscles over the sciatic nerve in the buttocks and to decrease pain and inflammation, use the ureters as a Process Center.

- Place one hand on the middle of the buttocks.
- Place the second hand behind the low back, on the ureters.

This hand placement configuration can be continued for as long as the pain and movement disorder improve.

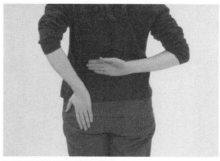

BUTTOCKS AND URETERS

STEP 2

While the sciatic nerve continues to heal and the symptoms subside, consider continuing with the following self-healing process.

- Read about the Process Centers as outlined and explained in Chapter 6.
- Choose the Process Centers you want to explore and read about them in Part II.
- Place one hand over the middle of the buttocks, over the sciatic nerve.
- Place the second hand on the Process Center of your choice.

You can continue this process for as long as you wish. There are no contraindications; there are no precautions.

SHIN
Pain and Inflammation; "Shin Splints"

Shin splints can be a nuisance and can cause a lot of pain. Shin splints are an inflammation of the periosteum of the tibia bone. Often there is a soft tissue problem (called fasciaitis) of the interosseous membrane between the tibia and fibula bones. Occasionally there are one or more bone bruises of the tibia, causing severe pain. A bone bruise has been defined as a *micro-trabecular fracture,* and can be diagnosed also with high density MRI.

Shin splints are common in athletes and runners. They are also common in persons with flat feet, and occasionally in persons with very high arches.

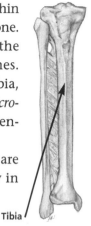

Tibia

STEP 1

To decrease the pain and inflammation of shins:

- Place one hand on the front of the tibia.
- Place the second hand behind the low back, on the ureters.

Hold this hand placement for at least one hour in mild cases. Maintain for longer if pain continues to subside. Maintain this hand placement for three to five hours (does not need to be consecutive) for more severe and long-term problems.

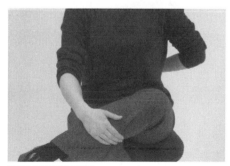

SHIN AND URETERS

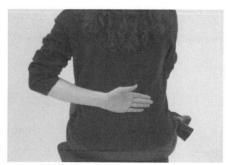

SHIN AND URETERS (REAR VIEW)

STEP 2

If pain and inflammation has decreased yet discomfort remains while running, consider continuing with the following treatment.

- Read about the parietals as a Process Center in this book.
- Place one hand on the shin.
- Place the second hand on the top of the head, over the parietals.

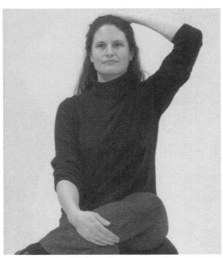

Practice running. As long as discomfort continues to decrease, continue with this treatment.

SHIN AND PARIETALS

STEP 3

While the shin continues to heal and the symptoms subside, consider continuing with the following self-healing process for the shin.

- Read about the Process Centers as outlined and explained in Chapter 6.
- Choose the Process Centers you want to explore and read about them in Part II.
- Place one hand over the shin.
- Place the second hand on the Process Center of your choice.

You can continue this process for as long as you wish. There are no contraindications; there are no precautions.

SHOULDER
Pain; Tendonitis; Bursitis; Pre- and Post-Shoulder Surgery; Fracture

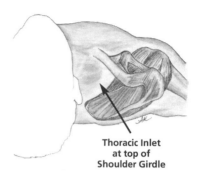

The shoulder is a vulnerable area. We use it often to our disadvantage. We lift, push, shove, hold, elevate, mobilize, and do other remarkable feats with our arms. The stable place for actions and activities with our arms is the shoulder. The shoulder girdle contains several joints. It includes the glenohumeral joint, the acromioclavicular joint, the scapulothoracic joint, and the

Thoracic Inlet at top of Shoulder Girdle

sternoclavicular joint. It also includes the front and back rib joints of the first four ribs.

So many persons complain of shoulder pain, yet they must continue to work with their hands and arms. For such people, even putting away the dishes on the top shelves can be agonizing. Shoveling snow can cause discomfort for days. Raking leaves, playing basketball—all activities we want and need to continue with—can make the shoulder region hurt more.

In order to get really good results with Neurofascial Process for the shoulder region, contact must be accurate over the whole region. This means: if you know where the problem is, place your hand over that area. If you are not certain because the total shoulder girdle region hurts, you will need to contact the whole front, back, side and top of the shoulder girdle.

If you are suffering from a swollen arm, the problem might be in the thoracic inlet region. Fluids in the arm drain into the thoracic inlet. Occasionally there are diagnoses such as *thoracic outlet syndrome* or *reflex sympathetic dystrophy*. These are often thoracic inlet problems. Therefore, in working with the shoulder, be sure to cover the top of the shoulder girdle, the region of the thoracic inlet.

Brachial Plexus   **Clavipectoral Fascia**   **Glenohumeral Joint**

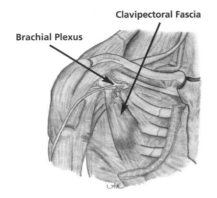
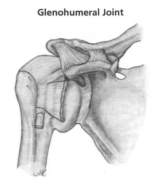

At the front part of the shoulder girdle is the clavipectoral region, where the clavicle and pectorals are centered. In this area is the brachial plexus. Compression of the brachial plexus at the clavipectoral region is a common cause of pain or numbness. This pain can be local, at the shoulder, or running down the arm, causing discomfort throughout the arm, and even causing tingling in the fingers. Be sure to cover this area whenever you treat the shoulder.

The glenohumeral joint itself has many ligaments, a capsule, synovial membrane, and other tissues. Contact the total region well, and your results will be excellent.

STEP 1

Often there is inflammation in and around the shoulder joint. Use the ureters for alleviation of swelling, heat, pain, and redness around the shoulder.

- Place one hand or more to contact the shoulder. Consider all aspects of the shoulder girdle: top, front, side, and back.
- Place the second hand behind the low back, on the ureters.

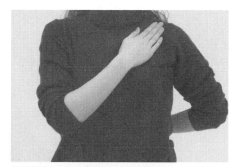

CLAVIPECTORAL AND URETERS

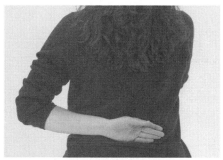

CLAVIPECTORAL AND URETERS (REAR VIEW)

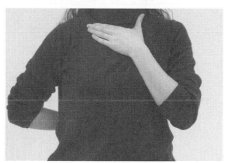

THORACIC INLET AND URETERS

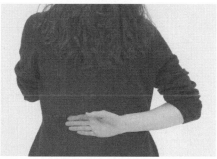

THORACIC INLET AND URETERS (REAR VIEW)

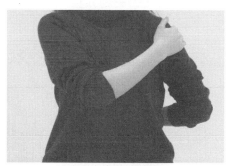

LATERAL SHOULDER AND URETERS

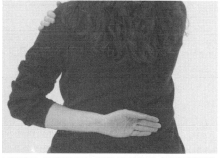

LATERAL SHOULDER AND URETERS (REAR VIEW)

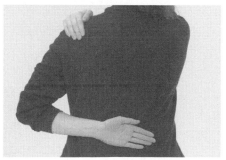

BACK OF SHOULDER AND URETERS

STEP 2

Wear and tear on the joints of the shoulder is common. Use the heart as a Process Center for healing.

- Place one hand over the shoulder joint.
- Place the second hand over the heart.

For acute problems, maintain this position for one hour or more. For long-term and severe problems, you can maintain these hand placements for up to twenty hours or more (does not need to be consecutive), as the arm becomes less painful, looser, and more user-friendly.

STEP 3

While the shoulder joint and shoulder girdle continue to heal and the symptoms subside, consider continuing with the following self-healing process for the shoulder joint and shoulder girdle.

All of the Process Centers are important. You will benefit from each one. You will be able to do more with your arm.

- Read about the Process Centers as outlined and explained in Chapter 6.
- Choose the Process Centers you want to explore and read about them in Part II.
- Place one hand on the shoulder joint and shoulder girdle. You may want to have other persons help you with hand placements, so that you can cover the total shoulder girdle region: front, back, top and side. Try to be accurate, and cover all areas as shown in the photographs.
- Place the second hand on the Process Center of your choice.

You can continue this process for as long as you wish. There are no contraindications; there are no precautions.

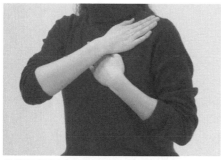

CLAVIPECTORAL AND HEART

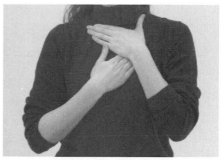

THORACIC INLET AND HEART

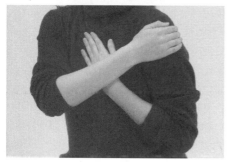

LATERAL SHOULDER AND HEART

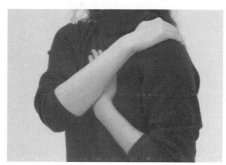

BACK OF SHOULDER AND HEART

SPINE
Pain; Spinal Cord Trauma

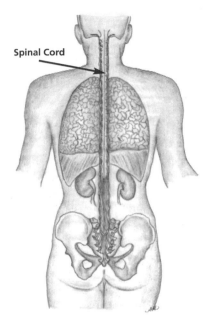

Spinal Cord

Often spinal pain and problems are named for the region of the problem. For example: "low back pain"; "cervical pain"; "cervical syndrome"; "neck pain."

If you are searching for a treatment for the low back or neck, please read the relevant sections (presented earlier).

When the entire spine hurts, use the following treatment to cover any and all regions of the spine.

If you have been the victim of trauma, in a car accident or have experienced a fall or athletic injury, often your injury is labeled a "spinal cord injury." Indeed, your spinal cord may be involved. I recommend, however, no matter how bad the injury—even if there is paralysis—that you try this approach. You can do so immediately after the injury. As long as you do not move the spine, you can use this approach even if the injury is acute and the spine appears severed or stretched or compressed. There are no precautions or contraindications. You can utilize this approach for all persons with spinal cord injuries, whether acute or long-term, whether mild or severe. Don't ever give up hope!

STEP 1

When there is an acute injury to the spine, there is swelling, inflammation, and often heat. Muscles may be torn; the blood vessels may be injured; the nerves throughout the region may be stretched, compressed, torn and even in shock. Use the ureters as a Process Center to address the spine under the circumstances of pain, inflammation, shock, and acute or chronic illness.

- Place one hand touching the area or areas of the spine involved.
- Place the second hand behind the low back, on the ureters.

When the injury is acute and severe, maintain contact for at least five hours (does not need to be consecutive). Give Neurofascial Process a chance. Even if all appears hopeless, at the very least pain and inflammation will subside, and healing will occur faster. If there appears to be an improvement, maintain contact with the ureters for up to a total of twenty hours or more (does not need to be consecutive).

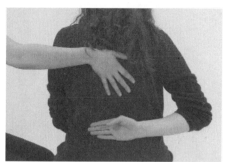

SPINE AND URETERS

When the injury or pain is long-term, start with five hours contact with the ureters. If there are changes in discomfort, movement, other circumstances, continue until all changes reach a plateau and come to a halt.

STEP 2

After treatment with the ureters, when pain and inflammation have decreased, and range of movement has perhaps increased, use the heart for healing.

- Place one hand on the involved area of the spine.
- Place the second hand on the heart.

Maintain contact for as long as required. The spine is a complex region of the body. It may require a lot of healing. Continue with contact as long as the symptoms are decreasing, and as long as there are indications of an increasing range of motion.

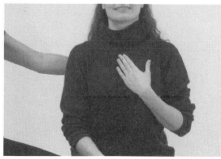

SPINE AND HEART

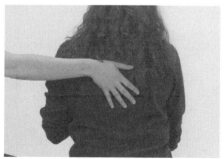

SPINE AND HEART (REAR VIEW)

Even if surgery has been recommended or you are paralyzed and have been given no hope of improvement, Neurofascial Process is still worth a try. It is less costly than surgery, less misery-causing than doing nothing, less dangerous than taking medications and other substances. When you are feeling the most hopeless, give it a chance: at least a total of five hours. If you perceive *any* changes in *any* signs or symptoms, give it another five hours.

While the spine continues to heal, and the symptoms are subsiding, consider continuing with the following self-healing process for the spine.

- Read about the Process Centers as outlined and explained in Chapter 6. All of the Process Centers are important. You will benefit from each one. Your spine will continue to heal: pain, function, and range of movement may all be transformed.

- Choose the Process Centers you want to explore and read about them in Part II.

- Place one hand over the spine. Try to be as precise as possible regarding the area of the spine that is involved, or else cover all areas of the spine where there is pain. You may want to have other persons help you with hand placements, so that you can cover all the relevant regions of the spine.

- Place the second hand on the Process Center of your choice.

You can continue this process for as long as you wish. There are no contraindications; there are no precautions.

SPLEEN
Immune System Problems; Autoimmune Disorders;
Illness in General

The spleen, together with other organs and structures in the body, is responsible for production of antibodies. Therefore, it is extremely important in all illness, as well as immune system and autoimmune problems.

When you are interested in improving the immune system, for whatever reason, follow the following protocol. Even if you are suffering from a degenerative disease, do not give up hope.

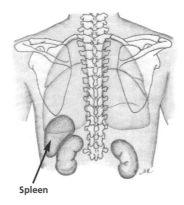

Spleen

STEP 1

• Place one hand on the spleen.

• Place the second hand behind the low back, on the ureters.

If you are very ill, maintain this contact for at least ten hours (does not need to be consecutive). Continue as long as your condition continues to improve. You will know you are improving if you are sleeping better; moving better; if you are less stiff and full of pain; more alert and more capable of handling daily activities.

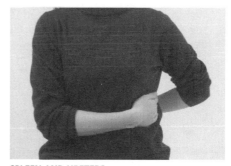

SPLEEN AND URETERS

STEP 2

- Place one hand on the spleen, as pictured in Step 1.
- Place the second hand behind the low back, at the level of the bottom ribs, on the kidneys.

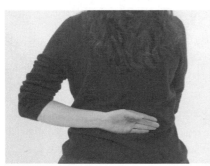

SPLEEN AND KIDNEYS

This connection will also take a long time, several hours. With a longer time there is more opportunity for healing and recovery.

Over time you may experience less toxicity, less fear, more movement, less pain, and an improvement in your general health.

STEP 3

It is often important to make a connection between the spleen and the liver. Often there is a great deal of toxicity. If the liver is congested, its failure to eliminate toxins may be part of the reason why the spleen became ill. If the liver is healthy, it will be able to purify some of the toxins within the spleen, which must be pure in order to produce antibodies. When your spleen is not healthy, and when it cannot produce an adequate amount of antibodies, you are immune deficient.

- Place one hand on the spleen.
- Place the second hand on the liver.

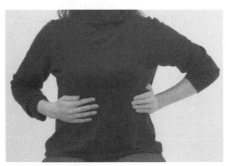

SPLEEN AND LIVER

This may also be a long process. Perhaps you have already performed twenty hours of Neurofascial Process between the spleen and the liver, yet you are feeling more health and vibrancy than you have enjoyed for many years. Even if you are feeling better, continue.

STEP 4

Here is another option for healing the spleen and for correcting immune disorders: Perform Neurofascial Process between the spleen and the major lymph nodes.

- Place one hand on the spleen.
- Place the second hand on the major lymph nodes as follows: both sides of the neck; over the heart; under the armpit; in the groin and front of the hip; over all areas of the abdomen. You can use family and friends in order to cover many lymph nodes simultaneously.

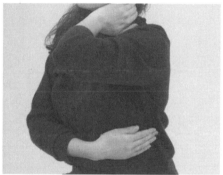

SPLEEN AND NECK

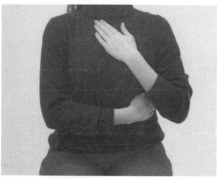

SPLEEN AND HEART

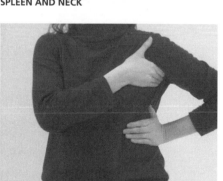

SPLEEN AND UNDER ARMPITS

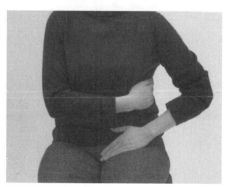

SPLEEN AND GROIN

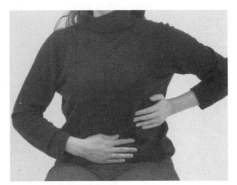

SPLEEN AND ABDOMEN

STEP 5

While you are beginning to heal and the symptoms are subsiding, consider continuing with the following self-healing processes for the as long as it takes!

All of the Process Centers are important. You will benefit from each one. You will continue to heal: pain, function, and movement will all be transformed.

- Read about the Process Centers as outlined and explained in Chapter 6.

- Choose the Process Centers you want to explore and read about them in Part II.

- Place the second hand on the Process Center of your choice.

You can continue this process for as long as you wish. There are no contraindications; there are no precautions.

STRESS
Psycho-Social, Emotional, Mental, Cognitive, Personal, Spiritual Disorders

The person who feels stress in their life (who doesn't?) should perhaps consider reading the first portion of this book. Read about the Process Centers. Learn about the different bodies. Perhaps read about the history of this author, who has faced trauma and learned to love life.

In working with stress it is first important to drain excessive stress-causing energies.

STEP 1

- Read about the following Process Centers in this book: kidneys; the limbic system; heart; the Emotional Body; the Mental Body.

- Perform Neurofascial Process connecting each of these Process Centers to the ureters.

- Place one hand behind the low back, on the ureters.

- Place the second hand over each of the following regions: kidneys; the bridge of the nose for the limbic system; heart; the Emotional Body; the Mental Body.

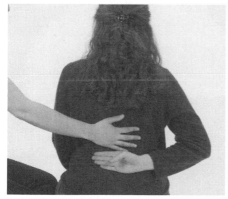
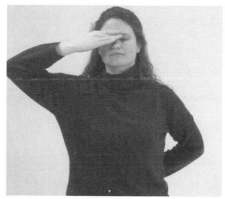

URETERS AND KIDNEYS   **URETERS AND LIMBIC SYSTEM**

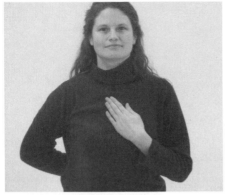

URETERS AND HEART

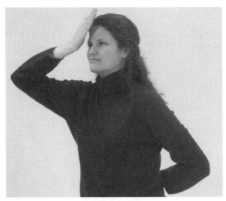

URETERS AND EMOTIONAL BODY

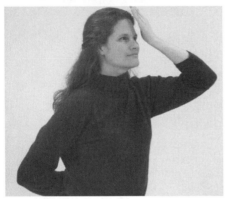

URETERS AND MENTAL BODY

STEP 2

- Once you have drained the above Process Centers in Step 1, consider a long-term approach to healing.
- Within this approach, read books on self-healing.
- Spend time with nature.
- Use your God-given talents to express yourself.
- Speak with people, about how you feel, what you think, who you are.

There are wonderful professionals who will listen, so that you can let go of pent up emotions, thoughts, and restlessness.

- Read about the Process Centers as outlined and explained in Chapter 6.

- Choose the Process Centers you want to explore and read about them in Part II.

- Place one hand on the above stress centers, one at a time or together. You may want to have other persons help you with hand placements, so that you can cover more stress centers simultaneously.

- Place a second hand over other Process Centers presented in this book. All of the Process Centers are important. You will benefit from each one. Your above stress centers will begin to function for you. You will notice healing: pain, behavior, and movement may all transform.

You can continue this process for as long as you wish. There are no contraindications; there are no precautions.

TEETH
Toothache; Periodontal Disorders; Abscess

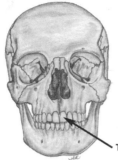

Teeth

Obviously, when you have a toothache you must go to a dentist. Yet perhaps you want to try an additional option to help you recover from the strain of tooth dysfunction. This approach will not cure tooth decay. Yet it can be enormously beneficial in reducing pain, inflammation, and often infection.

STEP 1

- Place one hand over your mouth, with good contact over the tooth or teeth that you want to influence.
- Place the second hand behind the low back, on the ureters, since the ureters is the Process Center for reduction of inflammation.

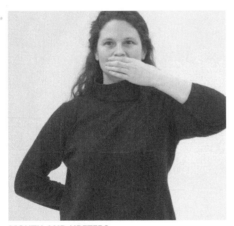

MOUTH AND URETERS

In case of inflammation and/or infection in your mouth, perhaps you can decrease some of the inflammatory process without requiring traumatic or invasive work. Perhaps visits to your dental hygienist will be more easily successful, when the hygienist needs to work less time on your mouth!

All of the Process Centers can be important in accomplishing this. You will benefit from each one. Your tooth or teeth will continue to heal: pain, inflammation, eating, chewing, and swallowing may become easier.

- Read about the Process Centers as outlined and explained in Chapter 6.

- Choose the Process Centers you want to explore and read about them in Part II.

- Place one hand over the tooth or teeth. Contact with gums is important for decrease in periodontal inflammation.

- Place the second hand on the Process Center of your choice.

You can continue this process for as long as you wish. There are no contraindications; there are no precautions.

THROAT
Sore Throat; Speech Impairments; Swallowing Problems

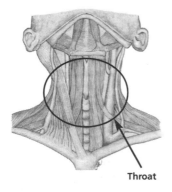

Throat

We use our throat for many purposes: talking, expressing emotions, communicating, eating, chewing, and swallowing. Problems in the throat include speech impairments such as poor verbal articulation, and swallowing problems such as drooling. Whenever there is *any* apparent discomfort with the throat, consider using Neurofascial Process.

STEP 1

If there is inflammation or infection, or just pain, use the ureters as a Process Center.

- Place one hand on the front of the throat with good contact.
- Place the second hand behind the low back, on the ureters.

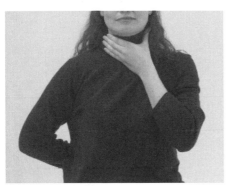

THROAT AND URETERS

For mild problems, maintain this contact for one hour. For moderate problems, maintain this contact for two hours. For severe and chronic problems, consider maintaining this contact for a total of three hours or more (in all cases, hours do not need to be consecutive).

STEP 2

After using the ureters for drainage and inflammation, consider continuing with the heart as a Process Center.

- Place one hand on the front of the throat.
- Place the second hand on the heart.

While your throat continues to heal, as you begin to feel better, or as your fever goes down, the range of movement in your neck movement is increased, or your speech and swallowing are improved—continue!

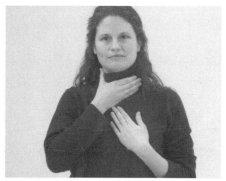

THROAT AND HEART

STEP 3

If you have a history of trauma, consider using the following Process Centers for continued healing: kidneys; the limbic system; liver; Emotional Body; Mental Body. What is considered trauma? Extensive mouth work at the dentist or orthodontist; surgery; fractures or direct contact to the throat; prolonged neck problems; whiplash or other injury from a motor vehicle accident.

- Read about the significance of these Process Centers in Chapter 6 and in Part II.
- Place one hand on the front of the throat.
- Place the second hand on the following Process Centers: kidneys; the bridge of the nose for the limbic system Process Center; the liver; the Emotional Body; the Mental Body.

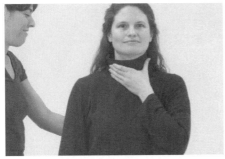

THROAT AND KIDNEYS

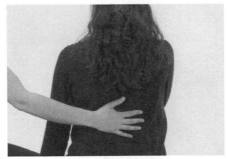

THROAT AND KIDNEYS (REAR VIEW)

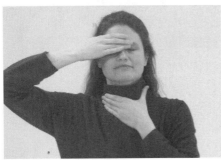

THROAT AND LIMBIC SYSTEM

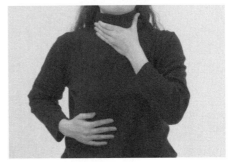

THROAT AND LIVER

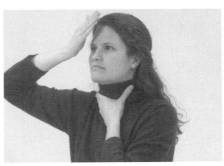

THROAT AND EMOTIONAL BODY

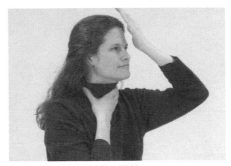

THROAT AND MENTAL BODY

STEP 4

Consider your history. The more it contains trauma or illness in your throat or mouth, the more self-healing you will want to perform.

All of the Process Centers are important. You will benefit from each one. Your throat will continue to heal: pain and inflammation will decrease, and eating, chewing, swallowing, and neck movements may become easier.

- Read about the Process Centers as outlined and explained in Chapter 6.
- Choose the Process Centers you want to explore and read about them in Part II.
- Place one hand on the front of the throat.
- Place the second hand on the Process Center of your choice.

You can continue this process for as long as you wish. There are no contraindications; there are no precautions.

WOMEN'S HEALTH ISSUES
PMS, Infections, Cramps, Bleeding, Other Problems

Women's health issues are a growing con-
cern in America. More incontinence prod-
ucts are sold to women for hyperactive
bladder than are sold for infants. Women
reach the age of thirty-five years old and
older, and realize that life is different from
before. Now when they run, play tennis,
make love, or even sneeze, many women
experience dribbling of urine and so require
those "diapers" for adults.

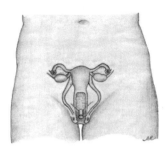

**Female Reproductive Organs
and Genital Region**

Why does this happen? Women experience trauma and surgery.
They use pills (birth control pills) that contain steroids meant to stop
the normal function of the uterus. They use tampons, IUDs, and latex
condoms with spermicide: all toxic to the internal organs. What can
they do about it? Become informed. Make choices. Learn to heal the
insides of the body, which have become inflamed and toxic because
of internal and external pollutants.

It is relatively easy to treat women for mild and moderate problems
of the genital region. When the problems are more severe, manual
therapy will add another dimension to self-healing with Neurofascial
Process.

STEP 1

To eliminate, or at least alleviate, inflammation and infections in the genital region, first use the ureters as a Process Center. Cover the total region of the uterus under the pubis bones, i.e. the region of the genitals at the pelvic floor. Help yourself stop itching, burning, pain, and other discomfort. Learn to enjoy life below the waist!

- Place one hand over the genital region. Cover the whole area.
- Place the second hand behind the low back, on the ureters.

If the problem is new or mild, perhaps one hour of working with the ureters will suffice.

The treatment will help all women, lessening signs and symptoms for several hours. Because there are no precautions or contraindications, this treatment can continue for up to a total of ten hours and longer (does not need to be consecutive).

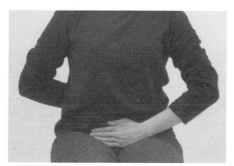 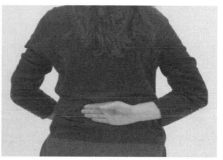

GENITAL REGION AND URETERS   **GENITAL REGION AND URETERS (REAR VIEW)**

STEP 2

Often women who have experienced trauma at the genital region need healing. The heart as a Process Center is remarkable for healing. Trauma can occur while giving birth, whether natural (vaginal) delivery or Cesarean section. Even being pregnant itself can be traumatic. Episiotomies are traumatic. So are many other forms of living.

Combine the genital region with the heart as a Process Center.

• Place one hand over the genital region, with good contact. Do not forget the pelvic floor.

• Place the second hand over the heart.

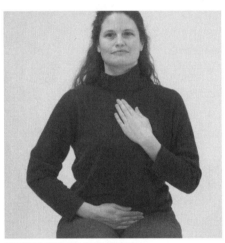

Maintain this contact for up to twenty hours (does not need to be consecutive), as long as symptoms continue to decrease.

GENITAL REGION AND HEART

STEP 3

Often sex has sinister connotations. Young women, many years ago, were afraid of sex itself. Today, the fear has different origins, yet fear is still there. Don't have sex because you might get pregnant. Don't have sex because your partner might have a sexually transmitted disease. Don't have sex because you are too young, not married, not pretty enough, etc.

Fears and anxieties about actions and activities related to the genital region are almost as severe as fears associated with coming of age. Should I get married? Should I have sex before I get married? Do I *want* to have children? *Can* I have children? How long can I wait before it is too late? What if I have children and then I no longer love my husband? What if I want children in spite of not having a husband? Will I ever be open enough to have sex? And more, and more, and more.

- Read about the following Process Centers in Chapter 6 and in Part II: the Emotional Body, the Mental Body, and the frontal center (forehead). Also read about the kidneys as the Process Center to affect fear.
- Place one hand on the genital region, with good contact.
- Then place the other hand on the following Process Centers, one at a time: the Emotional Body (the right side of the forehead); the Mental Body (the left side of the forehead); the center of the forehead; the kidneys.

Continue working with the genital region and these Process Centers for as long as you heal. Your itching will subside. Your burning and pain will decrease. You will walk with less tension at your hips. You will feel less discomfort when you experience emotions, thoughts, or activities related to the genitals and to sex. Your cramps will subside. You may feel more alive than you have in many years. Welcome to an era when womanhood is wonderful!

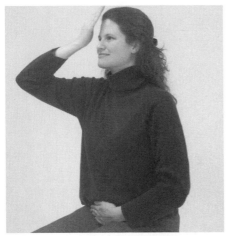

GENITAL REGION AND EMOTIONAL BODY

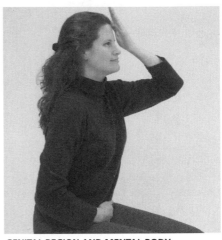

GENITAL REGION AND MENTAL BODY

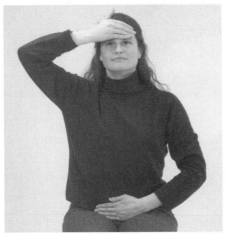

GENITAL REGION AND FRONTALS

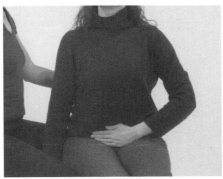

GENITAL REGION AND KIDNEYS

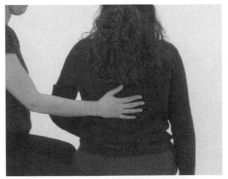

GENITAL REGION AND KIDNEYS (REAR VIEW)

STEP 4

Allow yourself to continue to heal the genital region. The philosophy is you don't know how good you can feel until you get there! While the genital region continues to heal and the symptoms subside, consider continuing with the following self-healing process for the genital region.

- Read about the Process Centers as outlined and explained in Chapter 6.
- Choose the Process Centers you want to explore and read about them in Part II.
- Place one hand on the genital region. Remember to cover the whole area from the pubis bone through the pelvic floor.
- Place the second hand on the Process Center of your choice.

You can continue this process for as long as you wish. There are no contraindications; there are no precautions.

WRIST
Pain; Carpal Tunnel Syndrome; Tendinitis

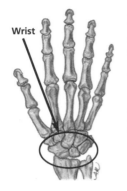

Wrist

In daily life, we need to perform many activities with our hands. We use our wrists to guide our hands, stabilize hand movements, and perform often heavy-duty tasks.

This self-healing approach can be utilized on all wrist pain and all wrist problems, no matter what the cause. Try this approach *before* you consider surgery. Use this approach immediately *after* surgery; healing will be enhanced. You can use this approach for chronic, acute, mild, and severe issues.

STEP 1

- Place one hand on the wrist. It is always best to cover the entire wrist. You may want assistance from family or friends for this.
- Place the second hand behind the low back, on the ureters.

Pain and inflammation will subside. Often when the problem is severe, or where there has been surgery in the past, or where the problem is long-term, treatment can continue for several hours (does not need to be consecutive). Maintain contact until all healing has come to a plateau.

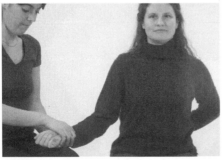

WRIST AND URETERS

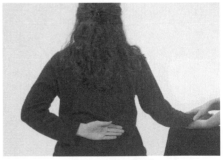

WRIST AND URETERS (REAR VIEW)

STEP 2

After using the ureters as a Process Center, consider utilizing the heart for further healing of the wrist.

- Place one hand on the wrist. It is always best to cover the entire wrist. You may want assistance from family or friends for this.
- Place the second hand on the heart.

Maintain contact on the wrist and heart while healing continues.

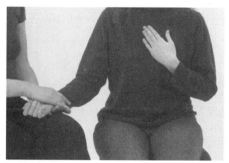

WRIST AND HEART

STEP 3

Consider your history. The more it contains injury to the wrist, the more self-healing you will want to perform.

All of the Process Centers are important. You will benefit from each one. Hand and wrist movements will improve and you will be able to grab more, pinch stronger, pull and push and lift better.

- Read about the Process Centers as outlined and explained in Chapter 6.
- Choose the Process Centers you want to explore and read about them in Part II.
- Place one hand on the wrist.

Place the second hand on the Process Center of your choice.

You can continue this process for as long as you wish. There are no contraindications; there are no precautions.

Summary

Neurofascial Process is a tool, a vehicle for healing. In conformity with the "Hippocratic Oath" that all physicians swear to, it can "do no harm." There are no precautions. There are no contraindications. There are very few people who cannot get some benefit from the processes outlined in this book. You only need time. Healing will come with patience and perseverance, but the desire to persevere will also come with the improvements you feel. When you feel you are healing, you will want to try more. When you try more, you will heal more.

Health insurance is expensive. Sickness is more expensive. Whatever *you* can do for your own self-healing, will provide enormous benefits. You will believe in your own self-healing capacity. We all self-repair, every minute, every second of every day. The ability to self-heal and self-correct is God's gift to all of us. Some of us need more time and effort, some less. You have all the time in the world—so use it! Believe in yourself. Believe in your ability to facilitate your own healing. The effect of self-healing is enormous. The effect of self-healing is hope!

Index

Self-control
    centers, 35
    limbic system and, 57
Self-healing, importance of, 203
Sex, 197
Sexual organs. *See* Genital region
Shin splints, 171–72
Shoulder problems, 173–77
Sinoatrial (SA) node, 24
Six Bodies, 17–20
Small intestine, 95
S1 vertebra, 119–24
Soul
    control and, 19
    manifestation of, 17
Speech impairments, 190–93
Spinal problems, 178–80. *See also*
    Low back pain; Neck pain
Spiritual Body, 18
    eyes and, 33
    heart and, 24
    liver and, 37
    lungs and, 25
Spleen
    immune system and, 181–84
    as Process Center, 29
Sports injuries
    knee problems, 151–56
    shin splints, 171–72
    spinal cord problems, 178
Sternoclavicular joint, 173
Stomachache, 95–109
Stress
    adrenals and, 32
    discharge of repressed emotional
        energies and, 21
    techniques for, 185–87
    thresholds, 32

Surgery
    ear, 136
    eye, 140, 141
    hip, 148
    knee, 152
    shoulder, 173–76
    spinal, 180
    wrist, 200
Swallowing problems, 190–93

Talus, 110–12
Teeth, 188–89
Tendinitis, 200–201
Thighs, upper, 38
Thoracic inlet, 173
Thoracic outlet syndrome, 173
Throat problems, 190–93
Thyroid, 31
Tinnitus, 134–36
Toothache, 188–89
Toxins, 28, 37, 99, 119, 128, 182

Ulcers, 95–109
Ureters
    abdominal ailments and, 96–98
    elbow pain and, 137
    knee problems and, 152–53
    low back pain and, 119, 128–30
    as Process Center, 28, 128
    prostate problems and, 166

Vision
    of children, 160
    fear and, 140
    problems, 139–42

Women's health issues, 194–99
Wrist problems, 200–201

About the Author

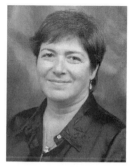

Sharon Giammatteo has had an incredible journey. After high school in Canada she studied in many locations, in many institutions. Her undergraduate degree is in Advanced Health Sciences and Medicine. Her diploma is in Physical Therapy. Her graduate degree is in Clinical Neuroscience. Her doctoral studies were in the field of manual and cranial therapies for neuromusculoskeletal dysfunction, with a focus on healing the neurological patient.

For years beginning in 1970, after graduation from Wingate Institute for Physiotherapy, the author traveled extensively to garner knowledge and skills in the fields of psychotherapy, manual therapy, cranial therapy, and rehabilitation. She has studied with leaders in their respective fields during the past thirty years. During that time, her goal was to develop techniques, concepts, and protocols. Her mission is, was, and will always be to contribute to recovery. With recovery a person can get on with life. A person can contribute to the services of mankind. A person can be on their path, unique and comprehensive for their own journey in life.

Sharon Giammatteo has an extensive background in the fields of traditional medicine, alternative medicine, and Western and Eastern philosophies. She has worked in hospitals, outpatient settings, schools and offices, in sports facilities, and on the field. Her work is with all client populations: children, adults, geriatrics; those suffering from conditions both acute and chronic; and with those needing attention to hands and feet and spine, brain and organs and orthopedics.

Much of her work was developed in order to alleviate pain and suffering. Some of her techniques were developed to help movement disorders and related disease and disability.

She began to develop Neurofascial Process as a system in 1981. She has developed almost all of the techniques in this book without help from others, although hundreds of colleagues and friends have used her approach and given her feedback. Thousands of her clients have used this treatment since 1981, and many more have used this approach while working with other practitioners.

Therapists all over North America and beyond are practicing Neurofascial Process. Doctors, chiropractors, naturopaths, nurses, speech pathologists, physical therapists, occupational therapists, and teachers are becoming familiar with this work.

Mothers and fathers treat their sons and daughters. Husbands and wives treat each other. Children and adults treat themselves.

This work has been performed at home, in the office, at school, in hospitals, in emergency rooms, in cars and airplanes and buses, in almost every possible setting.

This treatment has been used for all genders, ages, and nationalities. Every population has improved with this approach.

Sharing this work is the mission of this author.